kangaroo
mother care

A practical guide

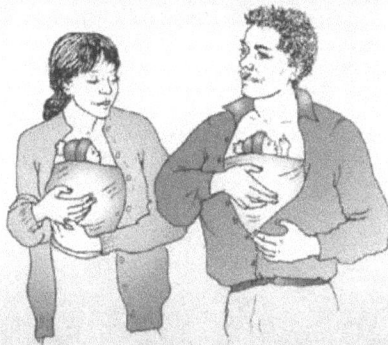

Department of Reproductive Health and Research
World Health Organization
Geneva

kangaroo mother care

A practical guide

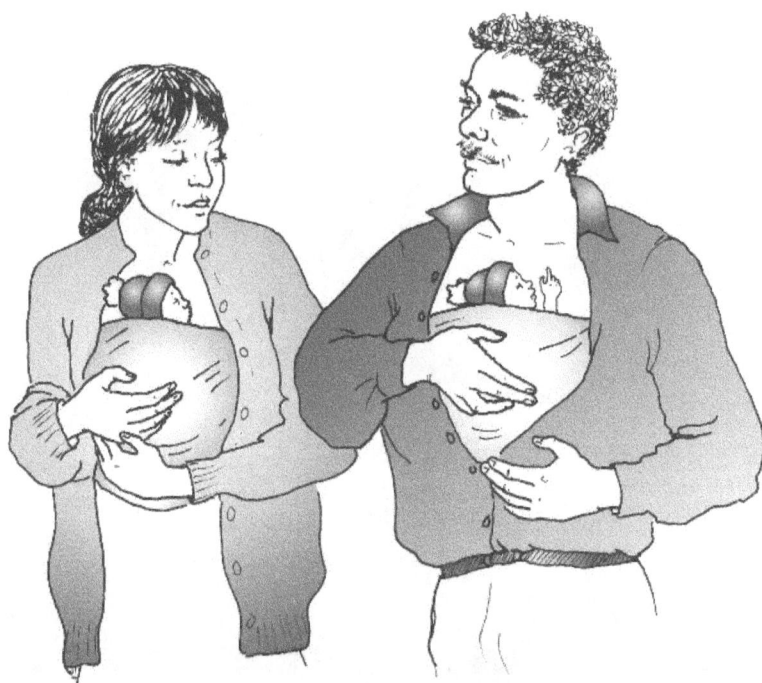

Department of Reproductive Health and Research
World Health Organization
Geneva

WHO Library Cataloguing-in-Publication Data

World Health Organization.
  Kangaroo mother care : a practical guide.

  1.Infant care - methods 2.Infant care - organization and administration
  3.Infant, Premature 4.Infant, Low birth weight 5.Breast feeding
  6.Guidelines 7.Manuals I.Title

  ISBN 92 4 159035 1   (NLM classification: WS 410)

Printed in France

TABLE OF CONTENTS

GLOSSARY

ABBREVIATIONS

ANNEXES 51

———✦———

TABLES

ILLUSTRATIONS

ABBREVIATIONS

LBW	Low birth weight
KMC	Kangaroo mother care
RCT	Randomized controlled trial
RDS	Respiratory distress syndrome

———✦———

GLOSSARY

Terms in this glossary are listed under key words in alphabetical order.

Age
    Chronological age: age calculated from the date of birth.
    Gestational age: age or duration of the gestation, from the last menstrual period to birth.
    Post-menstrual age: gestational age plus chronological age.
Birth
    Term birth: delivery occurring between 37 and 42 weeks of gestational age.
    Preterm birth: delivery occurring before 37 weeks of gestational age.
    Post-term birth: delivery occurring after 42 weeks of gestational age.

Birth weight

    Low-birth-weight infant: infant with birth weight lower than 2500g (up to and including 2499g), regardless of gestational age.

    Very low-birth-weight infant: infant with birth weight lower than 1500g (up to and including 1499g), regardless of gestational age.

    Extremely low-birth-weight infant: infant with birth weight lower than 1000g (up to and including 999g), regardless of gestational age.

Different cut-off values are used in this guide since they are more useful for clinical purposes.

Body temperature

    Hypothermia: body temperature below 36.5°C.

Growth

    Intrauterine growth retardation: impaired growth of the foetus due to foetal disorders, maternal conditions (e.g. maternal malnutrition) or placental insufficiency.

Milk/feeding

    Foremilk: breast milk initially secreted during a breast feed.

    Hind milk: breast milk remaining in the breast when the foremilk has been removed (hind milk has a fat content and a mean caloric density higher than foremilk).

    Alternative feeding method: not breastfeeding but feeding the baby with expressed breast milk by cup or tube; expressing breast milk directly into baby's mouth.

Preterm/full-term infant

    Premature or preterm infant: infant born before 37 weeks of gestational age.

    Preterm infant appropriate for gestational age (AGA): infant born preterm with birth weight between the 10th and the 90th percentile for his/her gestational age.

    Preterm infant small for gestational age (SGA): infant born preterm with a birth weight below the 10th percentile for his/her gestational age.

    Full-term infant small for gestational age (SGA): infant born at term with birth weight below the 10th percentile for his/her gestational age.

    Small baby: in this guide, a baby who is born preterm with low birth weight.

    Stable preterm or low-birth-weight infant: a newborn infant whose vital functions (breathing and circulation) do not require continuous medical support and monitoring, and are not subject to rapid and unexpected deterioration, regardless of intercurrent disease.

Note: Throughout this document babies are referred to by the personal pronoun "she" or "he" in preference to the impersonal (and inaccurate!) "it". The choice of gender is random.

1.
Introduction

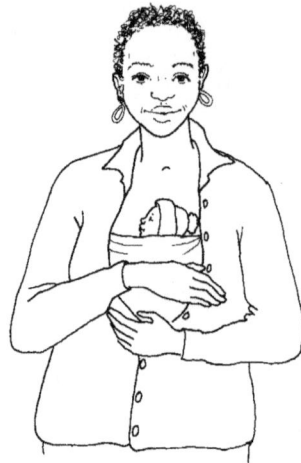

1.1 The problem – improving care and outcome for low-birth-weight babies

Some 20 million low-birth-weight (LBW) babies are born each year, because of either preterm birth or impaired prenatal growth, mostly in less developed countries. They contribute substantially to a high rate of neonatal mortality whose frequency and distribution correspond to those of poverty.[1,2] LBW and preterm birth are thus associated with high neonatal and infant mortality and morbidity.[3,4] Of the estimated 4 million neonatal deaths, preterm and LBW babies represent more than a fifth.[5] Therefore, the care of such infants becomes a burden for health and social systems everywhere.

In affluent societies the main contributor to LBW is preterm birth. The rate has been decreasing thanks to better socioeconomic conditions, lifestyles and nutrition, resulting in healthier pregnancies, and to modern neonatal care technology and highly specialised and skilled health workers.[6-8]

In less developed countries high rates of LBW are due to preterm birth and impaired intrauterine growth, and their prevalence is decreasing slowly. Since causes and determinants remain largely unknown, effective interventions are limited. Moreover, modern technology is either not available or cannot be used properly, often due to the shortage of skilled staff. Incubators, for instance, where available, are often insufficient to meet local needs or are not adequately cleaned. Purchase of the equipment and spare parts, maintenance and repairs are difficult and costly; the power supply is intermittent, so the equipment does not work properly. Under such circumstances good care of preterm and LBW babies is difficult: hypothermia and nosocomial infections are frequent, aggravating the poor outcomes due to prematurity. Frequently and often unnecessarily, incubators separate babies from their mothers, depriving them of the necessary contact.

Unfortunately, there is no simple solution to this problem since the health of an infant is closely linked to the mother's health and the care she receives in pregnancy and childbirth.

For many small preterm infants, receiving prolonged medical care is important. However, kangaroo mother care (KMC) is an effective way to meet baby's needs for warmth, breastfeeding, protection from infection, stimulation, safety and love.

1.2 Kangaroo mother care – what it is and why it matters

Kangaroo mother care is care of preterm infants carried skin-to-skin with the mother. It is a powerful, easy-to-use method to promote the health and well-being of infants born preterm as well as full-term. Its key features are:

❖ *early, continuous and prolonged skin-to-skin contact between the mother and the baby;*
❖ *exclusive breastfeeding (ideally);*
❖ *it is initiated in hospital and can be continued at home;*
❖ *small babies can be discharged early;*
❖ *mothers at home require adequate support and follow-up;*
❖ *it is a gentle, effective method that avoids the agitation routinely experienced in a busy ward with preterm infants.*

It was first presented by Rey and Martinez,[9] in Bogotá, Colombia, where it was developed as an alternative to inadequate and insufficient incubator care for those preterm newborn infants who had overcome initial problems and required only to feed and grow. Almost two decades of implementation and research have made it clear that KMC is more than an alternative to incubator care. It has been shown to be effective for thermal control, breastfeeding and bonding in all newborn infants, irrespective of setting, weight, gestational age, and clinical conditions.[10, 11]

Most published experience and research concerning KMC comes from health facilities, where care was initiated with the help of skilled health workers. Once a mother was confident in the care she gave her baby, she continued it at home under guidance and with frequent visits for specialised follow-up.

Evidence of the effectiveness and safety of KMC is available only for preterm infants without medical problems, the so-called stabilised newborn. Research and experience show that:

❖ *KMC is at least equivalent to conventional care (incubators), in terms of safety and thermal protection, if measured by mortality.*
❖ *KMC, by facilitating breastfeeding, offers noticeable advantages in cases of severe morbidity.*
❖ *KMC contributes to the humanization of neonatal care and to better bonding between mother and baby in both low and high-income countries.[12, 13]*
❖ *KMC is, in this respect, a modern method of care in any setting, even where expensive technology and adequate care are available.*
❖ *KMC has never been assessed in the home setting.*

Ongoing research and observational studies are assessing the effective use of this method in situations where neonatal intensive care or referral are not available, and where health workers are properly trained. In those settings KMC before stabilisation may represent the best chance of healthy survival. [14, 15]

This guide will therefore refer to KMC initiated at a health facility and continued at home under the supervision of the health facility (domiciliary KMC). KMC as described in this document recommends continuous skin-to-skin contact acknowledging that it might not be possible in all settings and under all circumstances. The principles and practice of KMC outlined in this document are also valid for intermittent skin-to-skin contact, provided adequate care is offered to LBW and preterm newborn infants when they are separated from their mothers. Such intermittent skin-to-skin contact has been shown to be beneficial,[16] if complemented by proper incubator care. Guidance on skin-to-skin care may be used for rewarming newborn infants with hypothermia or keeping them warm during transportation to the referral facility.[17]

1.3 What is this document about?

This document describes the KMC method for care of stable preterm/LBW infants (i.e. those who can breath air and have no major health problems) who need thermal protection, adequate feeding, frequent observation, and protection from infection.

It provides guidance on how to organize services at the referral hospital and on what is needed to introduce and carry out KMC, focusing on settings where resources are limited.

Evidence for the recommendations is provided[18] whenever possible. However, for many statements, especially those related to secondary procedures, sound evidence is not available as in many other fields of health care. In these cases, the text reports the experience of health professionals who have implemented KMC for many years, many of whom carefully revised previous versions of this document.

For breastfeeding counselling and support, readers should refer to *Breastfeeding Counselling: A Training Course -Trainer's Guide.*[19] For HIV and infant feeding, refer to *HIV and Infant Feeding Counselling: A Training Course -Trainer's Guide.*[20]

Management of medical problems of small babies is not part of this guide. Further guidelines can be found in textbooks or the WHO document *Managing newborn problems. A guide for doctors, nurses and midwives.*[56]

1.4 Who is this document for?

This text has been prepared for health professionals in charge of LBW and preterm newborn infants in first referral hospitals in settings with scarce resources.

It is not written for all potential care providers. Practical instructions (or protocols) adapted to the categories of health workers available in different settings should be prepared locally.

It is also aimed at decision-makers and planners at national and local levels. They need to know whether KMC suits the needs of their health systems, whether it is practical and feasible, and what is required to implement it successfully.

1.5 How should this document be used?

KMC guidelines have to be adapted to specific circumstances and available resources at national or local level. This document can be used to develop national and local policies, guidelines and protocols from which training material can be developed. This document cannot, as it stands, be used for training purposes. Other training material and activities, especially on breastfeeding support and counselling on HIV and infant feeding, are needed to acquire all the necessary skills. We hope that pre-service institutions will include those skills in their curricula.

2.
Evidence

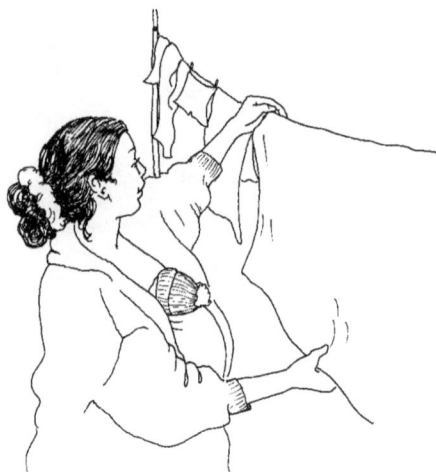

This chapter reviews the evidence on KMC, from both developing and developed countries, with regard to the following outcomes: mortality and morbidity; breastfeeding and growth; thermal protection and metabolism, and other effects. The experience with KMC has been reviewed by several authors,[12, 13, 16, 21, 22] and in a systematic review.[23] We also present evidence on the acceptability of the intervention for mothers and health-care staff.

While reviewing the evidence, regardless of the outcome, it became clear that it was important to highlight two essential variables: time of initiation of KMC, and daily and overall duration of skin-to-skin contact.

Time of initiation of KMC in the studies under consideration varied from just after birth to several days after birth. Late initiation means that the preterm/LBW infants have already overcome the period of maximum risk for their health.

Length of daily and overall duration of skin-to-skin contact also varied from minutes (e.g. 30 minutes per day on average) to virtually 24 hours per day; from a few days to several weeks. The longer the care, the stronger the possible direct and causal association between KMC and the outcome. Furthermore, when KMC was carried out over a long period of time, care was predominantly provided by the mother rather than the nursing staff or the conventional incubator.

Some other variables that might have affected the outcome of KMC are:

❖   *the position in which the baby was kept;*
❖   *the changes in the type and mode of feeding;*
❖   *the timing of discharge from the institution and the transition to home care;*
❖   *condition at discharge;*
❖   *the intensity of support and follow-up offered to mothers and families after discharge from the institution.*

Many other factors (e.g. social conditions, environment and health care, especially services offered for KMC) may be associated with the positive effects observed in KMC studies. It is very important to separate the effects of these factors from those deriving from KMC. Below, in reviewing the evidence, we try to address those additional factors.

No published study on KMC was found in the context of high HIV prevalence among mothers.

2.1 Mortality and morbidity

Clinical trials

Three published randomized controlled trials (RCT) comparing KMC with conventional care were conducted in low-income countries.[24-26] The results showed no difference in survival between the two groups. Almost all deaths in the three studies occurred before eligibility, i.e. before LBW infants were stabilised and enrolled for research. Infants weighing less than 2000g were enrolled after an average period of 3 -14 days on conventional care, in urban third-level hospitals. The KMC infants stayed in hospital until they fulfilled the usual criteria for discharge, as the control infants did, in two of the studies,[24, 26] while in the third study they were discharged earlier and subjected to a strict ambulatory follow-up.[25] The follow-up periods lasted one,[26] six[24] and twelve months,[25] respectively.

The RCT carried out in Ecuador by Sloan and collaborators showed a lower rate of severe illness among KMC infants (5%) than in the control group (18%).[24] The sample size required for that study was 350 subjects per group for a total of 700 infants, but only 603 babies were recruited. Recruitment, in fact, was interrupted when the difference in the rate of severe illness became apparent. The other controlled studies conducted in low-income countries revealed no significant difference in severe morbidity, but found fewer hospital infections and readmissions in the KMC group. Kambarami and collaborators from Zimbabwe also reported reduced hospital infections.[27] High-income countries report no difference in morbidity. However, it is notable that no additional risk of infection seems to be associated with skin-to-skin contact.[24-27]

Observational studies showed that KMC could help reduce mortality and morbidity in preterm/LBW infants. Rey and Martinez,[9] in their early account, reported an increase in hospital survival from 30% to 70% in infants between 1000g and 1500g. However, the interpretation of their results is difficult because numerators, denominators and follow-up in the KMC group were different from those in the historical control group.[28] Bergman and Jürisoo, in another study with an historical control group conducted in a remote mission hospital without incubator care in Zimbabwe,[14] reported an increase in hospital survival from 10% to 50% in infants weighing less than 1500g, and from 70% to 90% in those weighing between 1500 to 1999g. Similar results are reported from a secondary hospital in nearby Mozambique.[15] The difference in survival, however, may be due to some uncontrolled variables. The studies in Zimbabwe and Mozambique, conducted in hospitals with very limited resources, applied KMC very early on, well before LBW and preterm infants were stabilized. In the early study by Rey and Martinez, KMC was applied later, after stabilization. In both cases the skin-to-skin contact was maintained virtually 24 hours a day.

Charpak and collaborators, in a two-cohort study carried out in Bogotá, Colombia,[29] found a crude death rate higher in the KMC group (relative risk = 1.9; 95%CI: 0,6 to 5.8), but their results reverted in favour of KMC (relative risk = 0.5, 95%CI: 0.2 to 1.2) after adjustment for birth weight and gestational age. The differences, however, were not statistically significant. The two cohorts recruited in two third-level hospitals, showed many social and economic differences. KMC was also applied after stabilization and 24 hours a day. In a controlled but not randomized trial carried out in a tertiary-care hospital in Zimbabwe, there was a slight difference in survival in favour of the KMC infants, but this might have been due to differences in feeding.[27]

Conclusion

On balance the evidence shows that although KMC does not necessarily improve survival, it does not reduce it. After stabilization, there is no difference in survival between KMC and good conventional care. The hypothesis that KMC might improve survival when applied before stabilization needs to be further explored with well-designed studies. If such an effect on survival exists, it will be more evident and easier to demonstrate in the poorest settings, where mortality is very high.

As for morbidity, while there is no strong evidence of a beneficial effect of KMC, there is no evidence of it being harmful. In addition to the little evidence already published,[14, 15] some preliminary results on a small number of newborn infants with mild respiratory distress seem to confirm that very early skin-to-skin contact might have a beneficial effect.[30] A word of warning about discharge: KMC infants discharged during the cold season may be more susceptible to severe illness, especially lower respiratory tract infections, than those discharged during the warm season.[31] A closer follow-up is needed in such cases.

It should be noted that all the studies so far have taken place in well-equipped hospitals, yet arguably the most significant impact of KMC will be felt in settings with limited resources. There is an urgent need for further research in these settings. In the meantime, it seems that where poor conventional care is available, KMC offers a safe substitute, with little risk of raised morbidity or mortality.

2.2 Breastfeeding and growth

Breastfeeding

Two randomized controlled trials and a cohort study carried out in low-income countries looked at the effect of KMC on breastfeeding. All three studies found that the method increased the prevalence and duration of breastfeeding.[25, 26, 29] Six other studies conducted in high-income countries, where skin-to-skin contact was applied late and only for a limited amount of time per day, also showed a beneficial effect on breastfeeding.[32-37] The results of all these studies are summarized in Table 1.

It appears that KMC and skin-to-skin contact are beneficial for breastfeeding in settings where it is less commonly used for preterm/LBW infants, especially if these are cared for in incubators and the prevailing feeding method is the bottle. Other studies have shown a positive effect of skin-to-skin contact on breastfeeding. It could therefore be expected that the earlier KMC is begun and the earlier skin-to-skin contact is initiated, the greater the effect on breastfeeding will be.

Growth

The two-cohort study conducted in Colombia[29] revealed slower weight gain in KMC infants when compared with the control group, but the two cohorts also showed many social and economic differences. In the subsequent RCT[25] no difference in growth was observed at one year of age. In another RCT,[26] KMC infants showed a slightly larger daily weight gain while they were cared for in hospital, but in the overall period of study their growth did not differ from that of the control group. Similar results in terms of daily weight gain were observed in Zimbabwe.[27]

Table 1. The effect of KMC on breastfeeding						
Study	Author	Year	Ref.	Outcome	KMC	Control
RCT	Charpak et al.	1994	29	Partial or exclusive breastfeeding at:		
				1 month	93%	78%
				6 months	70%	37%
				1 year	41%	23%
RCT	Charpak et al.	1997	25	Partial or exclusive breastfeeding at 3 months	82%	75%
RCT	Cattaneo et al.	1998	26	Exclusive breastfeeding at discharge	88%	70%
	Schmidt et al.	1986	32	Daily volume	640 ml	400 ml
				Daily feeds	12	9
	Whitelaw et al.	1988	33	Breastfeeding at 6 weeks	55%	28%
	Wahlberg et al.	1992	34	Breastfeeding at discharge	77%	42%
	Syfrett et al.	1993	35	Daily feeds (34 weeks of gestational age)	12	12
	Blaymore-Bier et al.	1996	36	Breastfeeding at: discharge	90%	61%
				1 month	50%	11%
	Hurst et al.	1997	37	Daily volume at 4 weeks	647 ml	530 ml
				Exclusive breastfeeding at discharge	37%	6%

2.3 Thermal control and metabolism

Studies carried out in low-income countries[26] show that prolonged skin-to-skin contact between the mother and her preterm/LBW infant, as in KMC, provides effective thermal control and may be associated with a reduced risk of hypothermia. Fathers too can effectively conserve heat in newborn infants[38] despite an initial report of worse performance of males in thermal control.[39]

Heart and respiratory rates, respiration, oxygenation, oxygen consumption, blood glucose, sleep patterns and behaviour observed in preterm/LBW infants held skin-to-skin tend to be similar to or better than those observed in infants separated from their mothers.[40-42] Contact between mother and child has other effects also. For instance, salivary cortisol, an indicator of possible stress, appears to be lower in newborn infants held skin-to-skin.[43] This observation is consistent with the reporting of significantly more crying in full-term healthy infants 90 minutes after birth[44, 45] and in LBW and preterm infants at 6 months[33] of age when they are separated from their mothers.

2.4 Other effects

Kangaroo care helps both infants and parents. Mothers report being significantly less stressed during kangaroo care than when the baby is receiving conventional care. Mothers prefer skin-to-skin contact to conventional care[26] and report an increased confidence, self-esteem, and feeling of fulfilment, also in high-income countries. They describe a sense of empowerment, confidence and a feeling that they can do something positive for their preterm infants in different settings and cultures.[46-49] Fathers too said that they felt relaxed, comfortable and contented while providing kangaroo care. KMC thus empowers mothers and increases their confidence in handling and feeding their LBW and preterm infants. Tessier and collaborators, using data from the RCT conducted in Colombia, concluded that KMC should be encouraged as soon as possible after birth because it improves bonding and makes mothers feel more competent.[50]

KMC is acceptable to health-care staff, and the presence of mothers in the ward does not seem to be a problem. Most health workers consider KMC beneficial. They may think that conventional incubator care allows better monitoring of sick LBW and preterm infants, but they recognize that it increases the risk of hospital infections and it separates infants from their mothers. Health workers would prefer KMC for their own preterm/LBW infant.[26]

Lower capital investment and recurrent costs is yet another advantage of KMC and could bring about some savings to hospitals and health care systems in low-income countries. Savings may result from reduced spending on fuel, electricity, maintenance and repair of equipment[26] as well as possible reduction in staffing costs, since mothers provide the greater proportion of care. Compared with conventional incubator care, Ecuador[24] has reported lower costs per infant, in part associated with a reduced rate of readmission to hospital. This may partly be due to a shorter length of hospital stay in KMC infants, reported from both low [25-27] and high-income countries.[33, 35, 46] Capital and recurrent savings may be more substantial in tertiary than in first-referral and small facilities in low-income countries.

2.5 Research needs

More evidence of the advantages of KMC over other methods of care is needed, particularly on:

- ❖ *the effectiveness and safety of KMC before stabilization, in settings with very limited resources (i.e. without incubators and other expensive technologies);*
- ❖ *breastfeeding and feeding supplements in LBW infants less than 32 weeks of gestational age;*
- ❖ *simpler and reliable methods for monitoring the well-being of KMC infants, especially breathing and feeding;*
- ❖ *KMC in LBW infants weighing less than 1000g, and in newborn infants who are critically ill;*
- ❖ *KMC in very special circumstances, e.g. in very cold climates or in refugee camps;*
- ❖ *cultural and managerial barriers that may hinder the implementation of KMC, and interventions that may foster it, particularly in settings with very limited resources;*
- ❖ *the implementation of KMC for LBW and preterm infants delivered at home without the help of trained personnel and without the possibility of referral to the appropriate level of care.*

This last situation may well be the most important current source of perinatal and neonatal mortality and morbidity. The evidence about the benefits of KMC for LBW and preterm infants relates to those born and assisted in health facilities or who can benefit from careful follow-up at home, not to those delivered at home. Clear scientific evidence is needed to establish the safety and suitability of domiciliary KMC for babies born at home. However, there is no evidence that such care would be harmful or less safe than current practice. It might be reasonable, unless future research showed that other methods of home care were more effective, to recommend KMC for the home care of LBW and preterm infants born at home and who cannot be taken to hospital. Local culture and local activities to improve birth care at home should be taken into account if such a recommendation were issued.

3.
Requirements

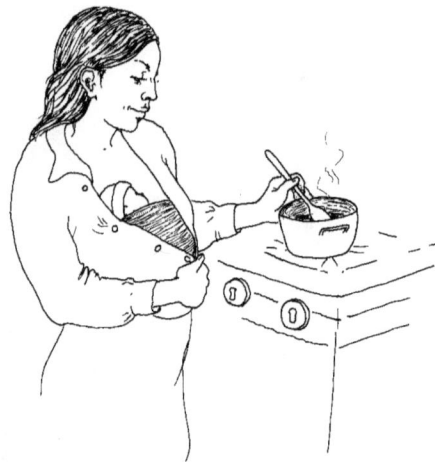

The most important resources for KMC are the mother, personnel with special skills and a supportive environment. The requirements described in this chapter are formulation of policy, organization of services and follow-up, equipment and supplies for mothers and babies, and skilled providers for the facilities. Some common constraints faced when implementing KMC, and possible solutions, are discussed in Annex III.

Very small newborn infants and those with complications are best cared for in incubators where they can receive the necessary attention and care. As soon as the general condition improves and the baby no longer needs intensive medical care, but simply warmth, protection from infections and adequate feeding to ensure growth, KMC can be the method of choice.

3.1 Setting

KMC can be implemented in various facilities and at different levels of care. The most common settings where such care can be implemented, are described below:

Maternity facilities

Small maternity units with several deliveries per day, these facilities are usually staffed by skilled midwives but often have no doctors and lack special equipment (incubators and radiant warmers) and supplies (oxygen, drugs and preterm formula) for the care of LBW and preterm newborn infants. If possible, such infants are transferred to a higher level of care; otherwise they are kept with their mothers and discharged early for home care. Hypothermia, infections, respiratory and feeding problems contribute to high mortality rates among those infants.

Referral hospitals

This category includes a wide range of special care units in district and provincial hospitals. A common feature is the availability of skilled personnel (specialized nurses and midwives, paediatricians, obstetricians, or at least experienced physicians) and basic equipment and supplies for special neonatal care. However, in reality, staff and equipment are often in short supply: competent physicians may be available a few hours per day only, small newborn infants are kept in large nurseries or wards, sometimes in contact with older patients. Mothers cannot stay with their infants and they have difficulty establishing and maintaining breastfeeding. Mortality may also be high for the same reasons. Abandonment may be a common problem.

There is a range of institutions between the two types of facility mentioned above, where skilled health workers can provide KMC.

3.2 Policy

Implementation of KMC and its protocol will need to be facilitated by supportive health authorities at all levels. These include the hospital director and the people in charge of the health care system at district, provincial and regional levels.

A national policy ensures a coherent and effective integration of the practice within pre-existing structures of the health system and education and training.

Preterm babies are best born in institutions that can provide the special medical care required for managing their frequent complications. Thus, when a premature baby is expected, the mother should be transferred to such an institution before birth. If this is not possible, very small babies or small babies with problems should be transferred there as soon as possible. The referral system should be organized in such a way as to guarantee the safety of the baby.

National standards and protocols need to be developed for the care of small babies, including those mentioned above, once they have overcome the initial problems. Standards must include clear criteria for monitoring and evaluation. These can best be developed by the appropriate professional groups with the participation of parents. Furthermore, local protocols will be easier to implement if national policies and guidelines are clearly set out.

Continuous monitoring and regular evaluation according to established criteria will help improve practice and design, and carry out research that may help refine the method.

Each health facility that implements KMC should, in its turn, have a written policy and guidelines adapted to the local situation and culture. Such policies and guidelines will be more effective if they are agreed on by consensus, involving all the staff, where possible, in developing local protocols based on national or international guidelines. The protocol should cover KMC as presented here, and should, of course, include follow-up. It could also be complemented by detailed instructions on general problems (e.g. hygiene of staff and mothers) or on problems commonly occurring in preterm infants (e.g. prevention and treatment of infection). After the introduction of the KMC protocol, monthly meetings with the staff will be useful to discuss and analyse data and problems, and to improve the protocol if necessary.

3.3 Staffing

KMC does not require any more staff than conventional care. Existing staff (doctors and nurses) should have basic training in breastfeeding and adequate training in all aspects of KMC as described below:

- ❖ *when and how to initiate the KMC method;*
- ❖ *how to position the baby between and during feeds;*
- ❖ *feeding LBW and preterm infants;*
- ❖ *breastfeeding;*
- ❖ *alternative feeding methods until breastfeeding becomes possible;*
- ❖ *involving the mother in all aspects of her baby's care, including monitoring vital signs and recognizing danger signs;*
- ❖ *taking timely and appropriate action when a problem is detected or the mother is concerned;*

- ❖ *deciding on the discharge;*
- ❖ *ability to encourage and support the mother and the family.*

Each institution should have a programme of continuing education in the area of KMC and breastfeeding. Nursing and medical schools should include KMC in their curricula as soon as possible.

3.4 Mother

Research and experience show that mothers like KMC once they have become familiar with it. KMC must therefore be discussed with the mother as soon as a preterm baby is born and offered to her as an alternative to the conventional methods when the baby is ready. Since KMC requires the continuous presence of the mother, it would be helpful to explain to her the advantages of each method and discuss with her the possible options regarding baby care. She must have time and opportunity to discuss the implications of KMC with her family, since this would require her to stay longer in hospital, continue the method at home and attend follow-up visits. If obstacles arise, talk about them and try to find solutions with the family before abandoning KMC. The mother must also be fully supported by the health workers to gradually take over the responsibility for the care of her small baby.

In theory it is possible to fully implement KMC with a surrogate mother (e.g. the grand-mother) but this is difficult to accomplish in practice.

3.5 Facilities, equipment and supplies

KMC does not require special facilities, but simple arrangements can make the mother's stay more comfortable.

Mother's needs

Two or four-bed rooms of reasonable size, where mothers can stay day and night, live with the baby, and share experience, support and companionship; at the same time they can have private visits without disturbing the others. The rooms should be equipped with comfortable beds and chairs for the mothers, if possible adjustable or with enough pillows to maintain an upright or semi-recumbent position for resting and sleeping. Curtains can help to ensure privacy in a room with several beds. The rooms should be kept warm for small babies (22-24°C). Mothers also need bathroom facilities with tap water, soap and towels. They should have nutritious meals and a place to eat with the baby in KMC position. Another warm, smaller room would be useful for individual work with mothers, discussion of private and confidential issues, and for reassessing babies. The ward should have an open-door policy for fathers and siblings.

Daily shower or washing is sufficient for maternal hygiene; strict hand-washing should be encouraged after using the toilet and changing the baby. Mothers should have the opportunity to change or wash clothes during their stay at the KMC facility.

Recreational, educational and even income-generating activities can be organized for mothers during KMC in order to prevent or reduce the inevitable frustrations of being away from home and in an institution. Noise levels should, however, be kept low during such activities to avoid disturbing the small babies. Mothers should also be allowed to move around freely during the day at the institution and, if possible, in the garden, provided they respect the hospital schedules for patient care and regularly feed their babies. The staff should use the long period in hospital (and the frequent contacts after discharge) to carry out other educational activities on infant and maternal health.

Mothers should be discouraged from smoking while providing KMC and supported in their anti-smoking efforts. Visitors should not be allowed to smoke where there are small babies, and the measure should be reinforced if necessary.

During the long stay at the facility visits by fathers and other members of the family should be allowed and encouraged. They can sometimes help the mother, replacing her for skin-to-skin contact with the baby so that she can get some rest.

Mothers, however, appreciate privacy while breastfeeding, taking care of their personal hygiene and during visits.

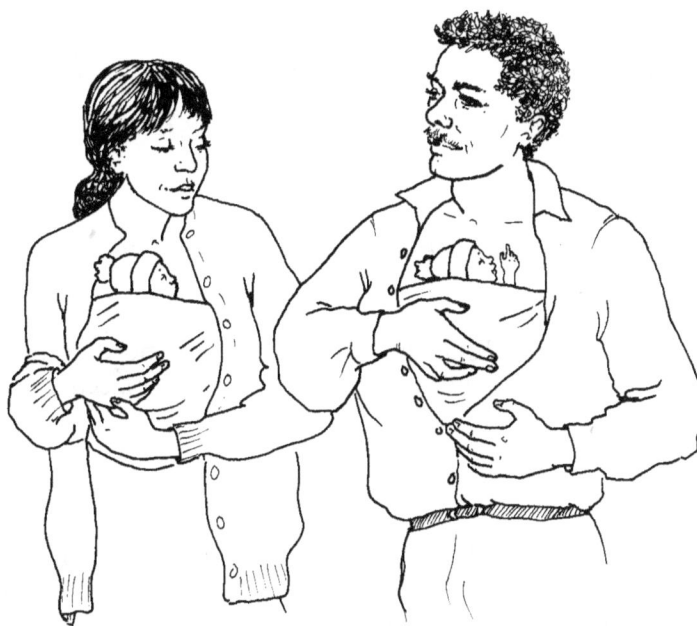

Fig.1 Holding the baby close to the chest

Clothing for the mother

The mother can wear whatever she finds comfortable and warm in the ambient temperature, provided the dress accommodates the baby, i.e. keeps him firmly and comfortably in contact with her skin. Special garments are not needed unless traditional ones are too tight.

The support binder

This is the only special item needed for KMC. It helps mothers hold their babies safely close to their chest (Fig.1). To begin with, use a soft piece of fabric, about a meter square, folded diagonally in two and secured with a safe knot or tucked up under the mother's armpit. Later a carrying pouch of mother's choice (Fig. 2) can replace this cloth. All these options leave the mother with both hands free and allow her to move around easily while carrying the baby skin-to-skin. Some institutions prefer to provide their own type of pouch, shirt or band.

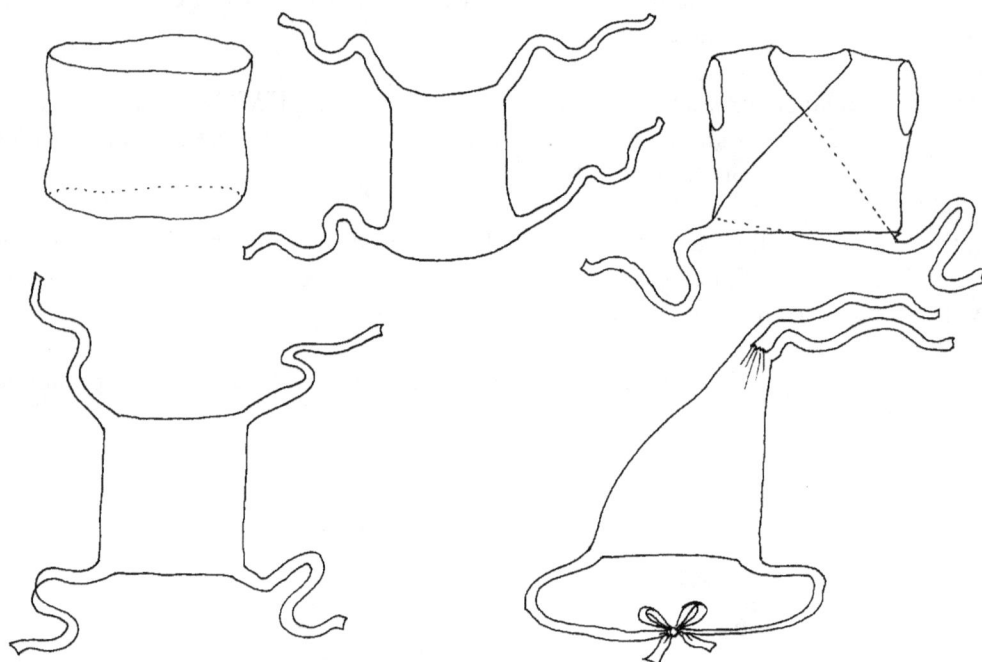

Fig.2 Carrying pouches for KMC babies

Baby's needs

When baby receives continuous KMC, he does not need any more clothing than an infant in conventional care. If KMC is not continuous, the baby can be placed in a warm bed and covered with a blanket between spells of KMC.

Clothing for the baby

When the ambient temperature is 22-24°C, the baby is carried in kangaroo position naked, except for the diaper, a warm hat and socks (Fig.3). When the temperature drops below 22°C, baby should wear a cotton, sleeveless shirt, open at the front to allow the face, chest, abdomen, arms and legs to remain in skin-to-skin contact with the mother's chest and abdomen. The mother then covers herself and the baby with her usual dress.

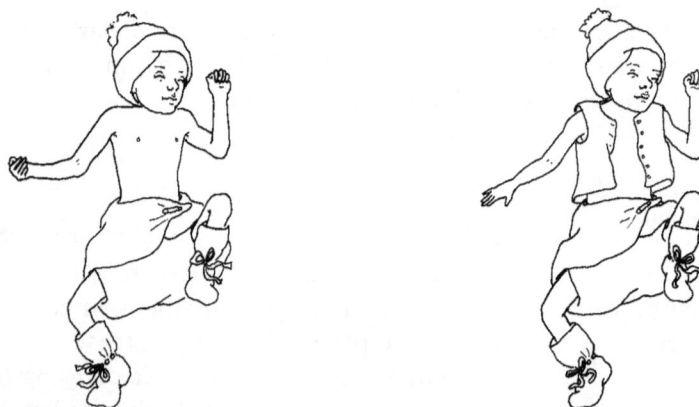

Fig.3 Dressing the baby for KMC

Other equipment and supplies

They are the same as for conventional care and are described below for convenience:

❖ *a thermometer suitable for measuring body temperature down to 35°C;*

❖ *scales: ideally neonatal scales with 10g intervals should be used;*

❖ *basic resuscitation equipment, and oxygen where possible, should be available where preterm babies are cared for;*

❖ *drugs for preventing and treating frequent problems of preterm newborn babies may be added according to local protocols. Special drugs are sometimes needed, but are not recommended in this guide. Treatment of medical problems is not part of this guide.*

Record keeping

Each mother-baby pair needs a record sheet to note daily observations, information about feeding and weight, and instructions for monitoring the baby as well as specific instructions for the mother. Accurate standard records are the key to good individual care; accurate standard indicators are the key to sound programme evaluation.

A register (logbook) contains basic information on all infants and type of care received, and provides information for monitoring and periodic programme evaluation. Annex I includes an example of the type of record sheet that can be used for this purpose and adapted to different settings. The data thus collected would also allow for regular calculation (e.g. quarterly and annually) of important indicators, listed also in Annex I.

3.6 Feeding babies

Mother's milk is suited to baby's needs, even if birth occurred before term or the baby is small. Breast milk is thus the best food for preterm/LBW infants and breastfeeding is the best method of feeding.[51, 52] Mother's milk should always be considered a nutritional priority due to the biological uniqueness of the preterm milk, which adjusts itself to the baby's gestational age and requirements.

In this guide only mother's milk is recommended for feeding her baby. Although pasteurized breast milk from another woman or the milk bank can be used, recommendations on pasteurization and milk banking are not included in this guide.

Breastfeeding preterm and LBW infants is a difficult task, and is almost impossible if the hospital and home environment are not supportive of breastfeeding in general. The staff need to be knowledgeable about breastfeeding and alternative feeding methods, and skilled in helping mothers to feed their term and normal weight infants, before they can effectively help mothers with LBW babies.

The ultimate goal is exclusive breastfeeding. KMC facilitates the initiation and establishment of breastfeeding in small infants. However, many babies may not breastfeed well at the beginning or not at all, and need alternative feeding methods. Therefore the staff should teach and help the mother to express breast milk in order to provide milk for her baby and to maintain lactation, to feed the baby by cup and to assess the baby's feeding. They should know how to assess the readiness of small babies for breastfeeding.

Hand expression is the simplest way to express breast milk. It needs no appliances, so a woman can do it anywhere at any time. Expressing breast milk by hand is recommended and described in this document.

Mothers need containers for expressed breast milk: a cup, glass, jug or a wide-mouthed jar.

Different kinds of breast pumps can also be used for expressing breast milk:

- *rubber bulb or syringe pumps;*
- *mechanical or electrical pumps, either hand or foot operated.*

These are particularly convenient for women who express breast milk several times a day over a long period. This is often the case when the baby is born long before term or requires prolonged intensive care (for more on breast pumps, see WHO breastfeeding counselling course[19]).

Cups, No. 5 to No. 8 French gauge feeding tubes and syringes are needed for feeding expressed breast milk or formula milk. Other tools such as droppers, syringes and teaspoons have been used instead of a cup. Traditional feeding devices, such as the "paladai" in India, have been shown to be effective.[53] A refrigerator also is needed for storing milk. Excess breast milk can be frozen.

Preterm formula must be available when breastfeeding is not adequate or for replacement feeding.

Health workers must be familiar with local harmful cultural practices, such as refusal to give colostrum or negative attitudes towards LBW and preterm infants ("they are ugly" or "they will not survive"). They should be trained to discuss such practices and attitudes with the mother and her family and find ways to overcome them.

3.7 Discharge and home care

Once the baby is feeding well, maintaining stable body temperature in KMC position and gaining weight, mother and baby can go home. Since most babies will still be premature at the time of discharge, regular follow-up by a skilled professional close to mother's home must be ensured. Frequency of visits may vary from daily at the beginning, to weekly and monthly later. The better the follow-up, the earlier mother and baby can be discharged from the facility. As a guide, services must plan at least 1 visit for every preterm week. Those visits can also be carried out at home.

Mothers also need free access to health professionals for any type of counselling and support related to the care of their small babies. There should be at least one home visit by a public health nurse to assess home conditions, home support and ability to travel for follow-up visits.

If possible, support groups in the community should be involved in the home (to provide social, psychological, and domestic work support). Mothers with previous KMC experience can be effective providers of this kind of community assistance.

4.

Practice guide

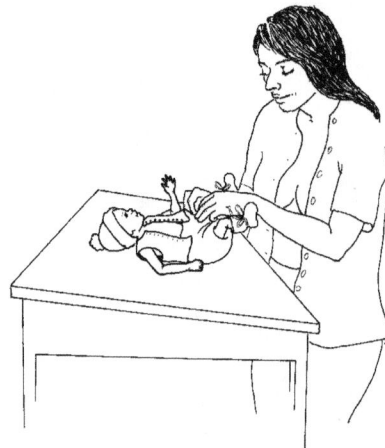

This chapter describes how to practice kangaroo mother care in the institution where a small baby has been taken care of and when to begin. It describes each component: thermal protection through the correct position, feeding, observing the baby, deciding when mother and baby can go home to continue KMC, and the follow-up needed to ensure adequate growth and to support the mother.

4.1 When to start KMC

When a small baby is born, complications can be expected – the more preterm and small for gestational age the infant is, the more frequent the problems are. Initial care for infants with complications is provided according to national or institutional guidelines. KMC will have to be delayed until the medical conditions improve. When exactly KMC can begin for those small babies must be judged individually, and full account should be taken of the condition and status of each baby and his mother. However, the mother of a small baby can be encouraged to adopt KMC very early on. The birth weight ranges below are given as a guide.

Babies weighing 1800g or more at birth (gestational age 30-34 weeks or more) may have some prematurity-related problems, such as respiratory distress syndrome (RDS). This may raise serious concerns for a minority of those infants, who will require care in special units. In most cases, however, KMC can start soon after birth.

In babies with birth weight between 1200 and 1799g (gestational age 28-32 weeks), prematurity-related problems such as respiratory distress syndrome (RDS) and other complications are frequent, and therefore require some kind of special treatment initially. In such cases the delivery should take place in a well equipped facility, which could provide the care required. Should delivery take place elsewhere, the baby should be transferred soon after birth, preferably with the mother. One of the best ways of transporting small babies is keeping them in continuous skin-to-skin contact with the mother.[10,54] It might take a week or more before KMC can be initiated. Although early neonatal mortality in this group is very high, mostly due to complications, most babies survive and mothers could be encouraged to express breast milk.

Babies weighing less than 1200g (gestational age below 30 weeks) incur frequent and severe problems due to preterm birth: mortality is very high and only a small proportion survive prematurity-related problems. These babies benefit most from transfer before birth to an institution with neonatal intensive care facilities. It may take weeks before their condition allows initiation of KMC.

Neither birth weight nor gestational age alone can reliably predict the risk of complications. Table 4 in Annex II shows how much the mean, and the 10th and the 90th weight percentiles, vary by gestational age for a population with mean birth weight of 3350g.[55] When exactly to initiate KMC really depends on the condition of the mother and the baby. Every mother should be told about the benefits of breastfeeding, encouraged and helped to express breast milk from the first day, to provide food for the baby and ensure lactation.

The following criteria will help determine when to suggest that the mother adopts KMC.

Mother

All mothers can provide KMC, irrespective of age, parity, education, culture and religion. KMC may be particularly beneficial for adolescent mothers and for those with social risk factors.

Carefully describe the various aspects of this method to the mother: the position, feeding options, care in the institution and at home, what she can do for the baby attached to her body and what she should avoid. Explain the advantages and the implications of such care for her and her baby, and always give the reasons behind a recommendation. Adopting KMC should be the result of an informed decision and should not be perceived as an obligation.

The following points must be taken into consideration when counselling on KMC:

❖ *willingness: the mother must be willing to provide KMC;*
❖ *full-time availability to provide care: other family members can offer intermittent skin-to-skin contact but they cannot breastfeed;*
❖ *general health: if the mother suffered complications during pregnancy or delivery or is otherwise ill, she should recover before initiating KMC;*
❖ *being close to the baby: she should either be able to stay in hospital until discharge or return when her baby is ready for KMC;*
❖ *supportive family: she will need support to deal with other responsibilities at home;*
❖ *supportive community: this is particularly important when there are social, economic or family constraints.*

If the mother is a smoker, advise her on the importance of stopping smoking or refraining from it in the room where the baby is. Explain the danger of passive smoking for herself, other family members and small infants.

Baby

Almost every small baby can be cared for with KMC. Babies with severe illness or requiring special treatment may wait until recovery before full-time KMC begins. During that period babies are treated according to national clinical guidelines.[56] Short KMC sessions can begin during recovery when baby still requires medical treatment (IV fluids, low concentration of additional oxygen). For continuous KMC, however, baby's condition must be stable; the baby must be breathing spontaneously without additional oxygen. The ability to feed (to suck and swallow) is not an essential requirement. KMC can begin during tube-feeding. Once the baby begins recovering, discuss KMC with the mother.

These general recommendations on starting KMC should be adapted to the situation of the region, health system, health facility, and individual. In settings with limited resources and when referral is impossible, the decision on when to start KMC during recovery should be weighed against the alternatives available for thermal control, feeding and respiratory support.

4.2 Initiating KMC

When baby is ready for KMC, arrange with the mother a time that is convenient for her and for her baby. The first session is important and requires time and undivided attention. Ask her to wear light, loose clothing. Use a private room, warm enough for the small baby. Encourage her to bring her partner or a companion of her choice if she so wishes. It helps to lend support and reassurance.

While the mother is holding her baby, describe to her each step of KMC, then demonstrate them and let her go through all the steps herself. Always explain why each gesture is important and what it is good for. Emphasize that skin-to-skin contact is essential for keeping the baby warm and protecting him from illness.

4.3 Kangaroo position

Place the baby between the mother's breasts in an upright position, chest to chest (as shown in Fig. 4a).

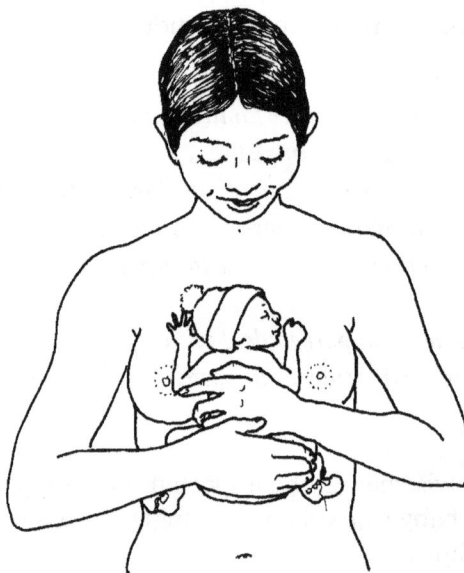

Fig.4a Positioning the baby for KMC

Secure him with the binder. The head, turned to one side, is in a slightly extended position. The top of the binder is just under baby's ear. This slightly extended head position keeps the airway open and allows eye-to-eye contact between the mother and the baby. Avoid both forward flexion and hyperextension of the head. The hips should be flexed and extended in a "frog" position; the arms should also be flexed. (Fig. 4a)

Tie the cloth firmly enough so that when the mother stands up the baby does not slide out. Make sure that the tight part of the cloth is over the baby's chest. Baby's abdomen should not be constricted and should be somewhere at the level of the mother's epigastrium. This way baby has enough room for abdominal breathing. Mother's breathing stimulates the baby (Fig. 4b).

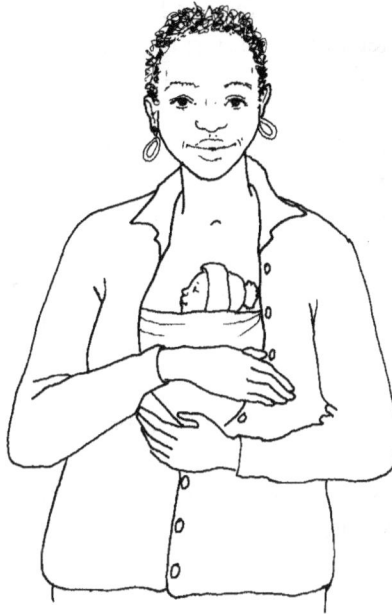

Fig. 4b Baby in KMC position

Show the mother how to move the baby in and out of the binder (Fig. 4c). As the mother gets familiar with this technique, her fear of hurting the baby will disappear.

Moving the baby in and out of the binder:

- ❦ hold the baby with one hand placed behind the neck and on the back;
- ❦ lightly support the lower part of the jaw with her thumb and fingers to prevent the baby's head from slipping down and blocking the airway when the baby is in an upright position;
- ❦ place the other hand under the baby's buttocks.

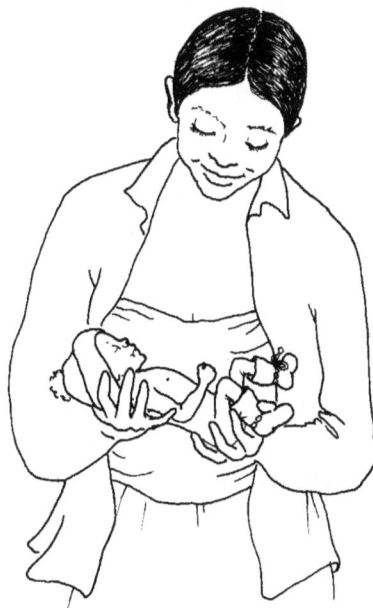

Fig. 4c Moving the baby in and out of the binder

Explain to the mother that she can breastfeed in kangaroo position and that KMC actually makes breastfeeding easier. Furthermore, holding the baby near the breast stimulates milk production.

Mother can easily care for twins too: each baby is placed on one side of her chest. She may want to alternate the position. Initially she may want to breastfeed one baby at a time, later both babies can be fed at once while in kangaroo position.

After positioning the baby let mother rest with him. Stay with them and check baby's position. Explain to the mother how to observe the baby, what to look for. Encourage her to move.

When introducing the mother to KMC also talk to her about possible difficulties. For some time her life will revolve around the baby and this may upset her daily routine. Moreover, a small baby at first might not feed well from the breast. During that period she can express breast milk and give it to the baby with a cup or other implements, but this will take longer than breastfeeding.

Encourage her to ask for help if she is worried and be prepared to respond to her questions and anxieties. Answer her questions directly and honestly – she needs to be aware of the limitations that KMC may put upon her daily activities as well as the benefits it can undoubtedly bring to her baby.

Experience shows that most mothers are very willing to provide KMC, especially if they can see other babies thriving. By sharing the same room for a long time, KMC mothers exchange information, opinions and emotions, and develop a sense of mutual support and solidarity. After a period of impotence and frustration during stabilization, they are empowered as the main caretakers of their infants and reclaim their maternal role from the staff.

4.4 Caring for the baby in kangaroo position

Babies can receive most of the necessary care, including feeding, while in kangaroo position. They need to be moved away from skin-to-skin contact only for:

- ❖ *changing diapers, hygiene and cord care; and*
- ❖ *clinical assessment, according to hospital schedules or when needed.*

Daily bathing is not needed and is not recommended. If local customs require a daily bath and it cannot be avoided, it should be short and warm (about 37°C). The baby should be thoroughly dried immediately afterwards, wrapped in warm clothes, and put back into the KMC position as soon as possible.

During the day the mother carrying a baby in the KMC position can do whatever she likes: she can walk, stand, sit, or engage in different recreational, educational or income-generating activities. Such activities can make her long stay in hospital less boring and more bearable. She has to meet, however, a few basic requirements such as cleanliness and personal hygiene (stress frequent hand-washing). She should also ensure a quiet environment for her baby and feed him regularly.

Sleeping and resting

Mother will best sleep with the baby in kangaroo position in a reclined or semi-recumbent position, about 15 degrees from horizontal. This can be achieved with an adjustable bed, if available, or with several pillows on an ordinary bed (Fig.5). It has been observed that this position may decrease the risk of apnoea for the baby.[57] If the mother finds the semi-recumbent position uncomfortable, allow her to sleep as she prefers, because the advantages of KMC are much greater than the risk of apnoea. Some mothers prefer sleeping on their sides in a semi-reclined bed (the angle makes sleeping on the abdomen impossible), and if the baby is secured as described above there will be no risk of smothering.

A comfortable chair with adjustable back may be useful for resting during the day.

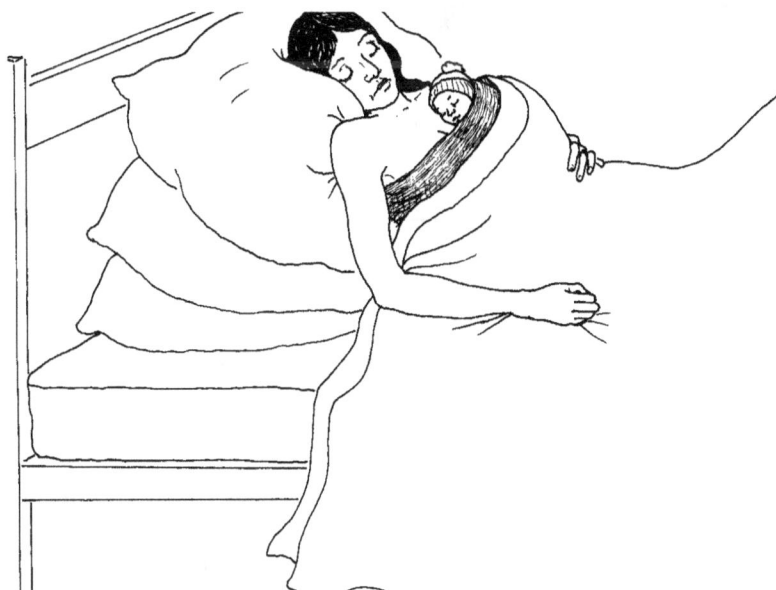

Fig.5 Sleeping and resting during KMC

4.5 Length and duration of KMC

Length

Skin-to-skin contact should start gradually, with a smooth transition from conventional care to continuous KMC. Sessions that last less than 60 minutes should, however, be avoided because frequent changes are too stressful for the baby. The length of skin-to-skin contacts gradually increases to become as continuous as possible, day and night, interrupted only for changing diapers, especially where no other means of thermal control are available.

When the mother needs to be away from her baby, he can be well wrapped up and placed in a warm cot, away from draughts, covered by a warm blanket, or placed under an appropriate warming device, if available. During those breaks family members (father or partner, grand-mother, etc.), or a close friend, can also help caring for the baby in skin-to-skin kangaroo position (Fig.6).

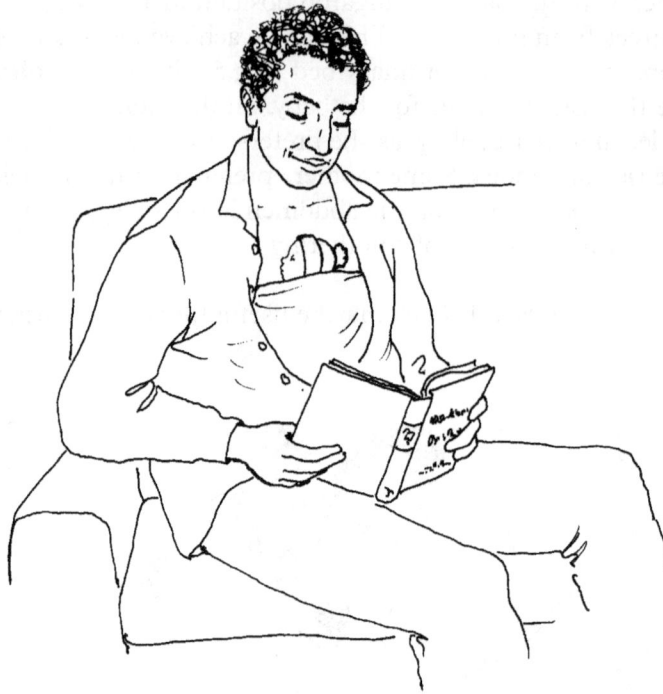

Fig. 6 Father's turn for KMC

Duration

When the mother and baby are comfortable, skin-to-skin contact continues for as long as possible, first at the institution, then at home. It tends to be used until the baby reaches term (gestational age around 40 weeks) or 2500g. Around that time the baby also outgrows the need for KMC. She starts wriggling to show that she is uncomfortable, pulls her limbs out, cries and fusses every time the mother tries to put her back skin-to-skin. This is when it is safe to advise the mother to wean the baby gradually from KMC. Breastfeeding, of course, continues. Mother can return to skin-to-skin contact occasionally, after giving the baby a bath, during cold nights, or when the baby needs comfort.

KMC at home is particularly important in cold climates or during the cold season and could go on for longer.

4.6 Monitoring baby's condition

Temperature

A well-fed baby, in continuous skin-to-skin contact, can easily retain normal body temperature (between 36.5°C and 37°C) when in kangaroo position, if the ambient temperature is not lower than the recommended range. Hypothermia is rare in KMC infants, but it can occur. Measuring baby's body temperature is still needed, but less frequently than when the baby is not in the kangaroo position.

When starting KMC, measure axillary temperature every 6 hours until stable for three consecutive days. Later measure only twice daily. If the body temperature is below 36.5°C, rewarm the baby immediately: cover the baby with a blanket and make sure that the mother is staying in a warm place. Measure the temperature an hour later and continue rewarming until within the normal range. Also look for possible causes of hypothermia in the baby (cold room, the baby was not in KMC position before measuring the temperature, the baby had a bath or has not been feeding well). If no obvious cause can be found and the baby continues to have difficulty in maintaining normal body temperature, or the temperature does not return to normal within 3 hours, assess the baby for possible bacterial infection.

If an ordinary adult-type thermometer does not record the temperature, assume there is moderate or severe hypothermia and act accordingly. Ways of identifying and treating hypothermia are described in detail in another WHO document.[10] Rewarming can be carried out through skin-to-skin contact.[17]

How to measure axillary temperature

- Keep the baby warm throughout the procedure, either in skin-to-skin contact with the mother and properly covered, or well covered on a warm surface;
- use a clean thermometer and shake it down to less than 35° C;
- place the thermometer bulb high up in the middle of the axilla; the skin of the axilla must be in full contact with the bulb of the thermometer, with no air pockets between skin and bulb;
- hold the infant's arm against the side of the chest gently; keep the thermometer in place for at least three minutes;
- remove the thermometer and read the temperature;
- avoid taking the rectal temperature since it is associated with a small but significant risk of rectal perforation.

Observing breathing and well-being

The normal respiratory rate of an LBW and preterm infant ranges between 30 and 60 breaths per minute, and breathing alternates with intervals of no breathing (apnoea). However, if the intervals become too long (20 seconds or more) and the baby's lips and face turn blue (cyanosis), his pulse is abnormally low (bradycardia) and he does not resume breathing spontaneously, act quickly: there is a risk of brain damage. The smaller or more premature the baby is, the longer and more frequent the spells of apnoea. As baby approaches term, breathing becomes more regular and apnoea less frequent. Research shows that skin-to-skin contact may make breathing more regular in preterm infants[41,58] and may reduce the incidence of apnoea. Apnoea appearing late may also indicate the beginning of an illness.

The mother must be aware of the risk of apnoea, be able to recognize it, intervene immediately and seek help if she becomes concerned.

> ### What to do in case of apnoea
>
> - Teach the mother to observe the baby's breathing pattern and explain the normal variations;
> - explain what apnoea is and what effects it has on a baby;
> - demonstrate the effect of apnoea by asking the mother to hold her breath for a short time (less than 20 seconds) and a long time (20 seconds or more);
> - explain that if breathing stops for 20 seconds or more, or baby becomes blue (blue lips and face), this may be a sign of a serious disease;
> - teach her to stimulate the baby by lightly rubbing the back or head, and by rocking movements until the baby starts breathing again. If baby is still not breathing, she should call staff;
> - always react immediately to a mother's call for help;
> - in case of prolonged apnoea, when breathing cannot be restarted through stimulation, resuscitate according to the hospital resuscitation guidelines;
> - if apnoeic spells become more frequent, examine the baby: this may be an early sign of infection. Treat according to the institutional protocol.

Once the baby has recovered from the initial complications due to preterm birth, is stable and is receiving KMC, the risk of serious illness is small but significant. The onset of a serious illness in small babies is usually subtle and is overlooked until the disease is advanced and difficult to treat. Therefore it is important to recognize those subtle signs and give prompt treatment. Teach the mother to recognize danger signs and ask her to seek care when concerned. Treat the condition according to the institutional guidelines.

> ### Danger signs
>
> - Difficulty breathing, chest in-drawing, grunting
> - Breathing very fast or very slowly
> - Frequent and long spells of apnoea
> - The baby feels cold: body temperature is below normal despite rewarming
> - Difficulty feeding: the baby does not wake up for feeds anymore, stops feeding or vomits
> - Convulsions
> - Diarrhoea
> - Yellow skin

Reassure the mother that there is no danger if the baby:

❖ *sneezes or has hiccups;*
❖ *passes soft stools after each feed;*
❖ *does not pass stools for 2-3 days.*

4.7 *Feeding*

Breastfeeding preterm babies is a special challenge.

For the first few days a small baby may not be able to take any oral feeds and may need to be fed intravenously. During this period the baby receives conventional care.

Oral feeds should begin as soon as baby's condition permits and the baby tolerates them. This is usually around the time when baby can be placed in kangaroo position. This helps the mother to produce breast milk, so it increases breastfeeding.

Babies who are less than 30 to 32 weeks gestational age usually need to be fed through a naso-gastric tube, which can be used to give expressed breast milk. The mother can let her baby suck her finger while he is having tube feeds. Tube-feeding can be done when the baby is in kangaroo position.

Babies between 30 and 32 weeks gestational age can take feeds from a small cup. Cup feeds can be given once or twice daily while a baby is still fed mostly through a naso-gastric tube. If he takes cup feeds well, tube-feeding can be reduced. For cup-feeding the baby is taken out of the kangaroo position, wrapped in a warm blanket and returned to the kangaroo position after the feed. Another way to feed a baby at this stage is by expressing milk directly into the baby's mouth. This way the baby does not need to be taken out from the kangaroo position.

Babies of about 32 weeks gestational age or more are able to start suckling on the breast. Baby may only root for the nipple and lick it at first, or he may suckle a little. Continue giving expressed breast milk by cup or tube, to make sure that the baby gets all that he needs.

When a small baby starts to suckle effectively, he may pause during feeds quite often and for quite long periods. It is important not to take him off the breast too quickly. Leave him on the breast so that he can suckle again when he is ready. He can continue for up to an hour if necessary. Offer a cup feed after the breastfeed, or alternate breast and cup feeds.

Make sure that the baby suckles in a good position. Good attachment may make effective suckling possible at an earlier stage.

Babies from about 34 to 36 weeks gestational age or more can often take all that they need directly from the breast. However, supplements from a cup continue to be necessary occasionally.

During this initial period the mother needs a lot of support and encouragement to establish and maintain lactation until the baby is ready to breastfeed. Primiparae, adolescent mothers, and mothers of very small infants may need even more encouragement, help and support during the institutional stay and later at home.

> ### *Discuss breastfeeding with the mother*
>
> - *Reassure her that she can breastfeed her small baby and she has enough milk;*
> - *explain that her milk is the best food for such a small baby. Feeding for him is even more important than for a big baby;*
> - *at the beginning a small baby does not feed as well as a big baby; he may*
>   - *tire easily and suck weakly at first*
>   - *suckle for shorter periods before resting*
>   - *fall asleep during feeding*
>   - *have long pauses after suckling, and feed longer*
>   - *not always wake up for feeds;*
> - *explain that breastfeeding will become easier as baby becomes older and bigger;*
> - *help her place and attach the baby in the kangaroo position.*

Breastfeeding

The kangaroo position is ideal for breastfeeding. As soon as the baby shows signs of readiness for breastfeeding, by moving tongue and mouth, and interest in sucking (e.g. fingers or mother's skin), help the mother to get into a breastfeeding position that ensures good attachment.

To start breastfeeding choose appropriate time - when the baby is waking from a sleep, or is alert and awake. Help the mother to sit comfortably in an armless chair with the baby in skin-to-skin position. For the first breastfeeds take the baby out of the pouch and wrap or dress him to better demonstrate the technique. Then put the baby into the kangaroo position and ask the mother to ensure good position and attachment.[19]

> ### *Help the mother to position her baby*
>
> - *Show the mother the correct position and attachment for breastfeeding;*
> - *show the mother how to hold her baby:*
>   - *hold the baby's head and body straight;*
>   - *make the baby face her breast, the baby's nose opposite her nipple;*
>   - *hold the baby's body close to her body;*
>   - *support the baby's whole body, not just the neck and shoulders;*
> - *show the mother how to help her baby to attach:*
>   - *touch her baby's lips with her nipple;*
>   - *wait until her baby's mouth is wide open;*
>   - *move her baby quickly onto her breast, aiming the infant's lower lip well below the nipple;*
> - *show the mother signs of good attachment:*
>   - *baby's chin is touching her breast;*
>   - *his mouth is wide open;*
>   - *his lower lip is turned out;*
>   - *a larger area of the areola is visible above rather than below the baby's mouth;*
>   - *sucks are slow and deep, sometimes pausing.*

Let the baby suckle on the breast as long as he wants. The baby may feed with long pauses between sucks. Do not interrupt the baby if he is still trying.

Small babies need breastfeeding frequently, every 2-3 hours. Initially they may not wake up for feeds and must be wakened. Changing the baby before the feed may make him more alert.

Sometimes it helps to express a little milk with each suck. If the breast is engorged, encourage the mother to express a small amount of breast milk before starting breastfeeding; this will soften the nipple area and it will be easier for the baby to attach.

Even if the baby is not yet suckling well and long enough (very preterm), offer the breast first, and then use an appropriate alternative feeding method. Do whatever works best in your setting: let the mother express breast milk into baby's mouth or let her express breast milk and feed it to the baby by cup or tube.

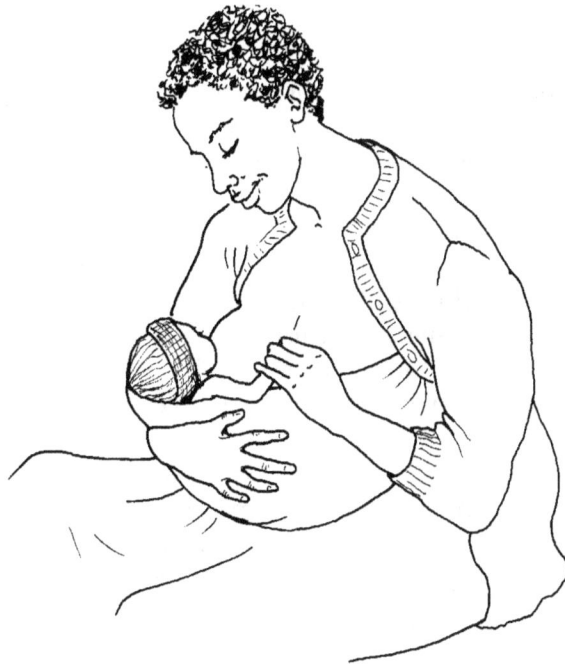

Fig.7 Breastfeeding in KMC

Give special support to mothers who breastfeed twins

- *Reassure the mother that she has enough breast milk for two babies;*
- *explain to her that twins may take longer to establish breastfeeding since they are frequently born preterm and with low birth weight.*

Alternative feeding methods

The baby can be fed by expressing breast milk directly into his mouth or giving expressed mother's breast milk or appropriate formula by cup or tube.

Expressing breast milk

Hand expression is the best way to express breast milk. It is less likely to carry infection than a pump, and can be used by every woman at any time. A technique to express milk effectively is described in the WHO breastfeeding counselling course.[19]

Show the mother how to express breast milk and let her do it. Do not express her milk for her. To establish lactation and feed a small baby she should start expressing milk on the first day, within six hours of delivery, if possible. She should express as much as she can and as often as the baby would breastfeed. This means at least every 3 hours, including during the night. To build up her milk supply, if it seems to be decreasing after a few weeks, she should express her milk very often for a few days (every hour) and at least every 3 hours during the night.

Mothers often develop their own style of hand expression once they have learned the basic principles. Some will express both breasts at the same time, leaning forward with a container between their knees and pausing every few minutes to let the sinuses refill with breast milk. Every mother will find her own rhythm, which is usually slow and regular. Encourage mothers to express breast milk their own way, providing it works for them.

If a mother is expressing more milk than her small baby needs, let her express the second half of the milk from each breast into a different container. Let her offer the second half of the expressed breast milk first. This way the baby gets more hind milk, which gives him the extra energy he needs and helps him grow better. If the mother can only express very small volumes at first, give whatever she can produce to her baby and supplement with formula milk if necessary.

Expressing breast milk takes time, patience and forward planning. Ask the mother to start at least half an hour before the baby's feed, irrespective of the method used. If possible, use freshly expressed breast milk for the next feed. If there is more milk than the baby needs, it can be stored in a refrigerator for up to 48 hours at 4°C.

Expressing breast milk directly into baby's mouth

Breast milk can be expressed directly into the baby's mouth, but the mother should first become familiar with expressing breast milk by hand.

The baby can be fed while in kangaroo position

- *Hold the baby in skin-to-skin contact, the mouth close to the nipple;*
- *wait until the baby is alert and opens mouth and eyes (very small babies may need light stimulation to be kept awake and alert);*
- *express a few drops of breast milk;*
- *let the baby smell and lick the nipple, and open the mouth;*
- *express breast milk into the baby's open mouth;*
- *wait until baby swallows the milk;*
- *repeat the procedure until the baby closes his mouth and will take no more breast milk even after stimulation;*
- *ask the mother to repeat this operation every hour if the baby weighs less than 1200g and every two hours if the baby weighs more than 1200g;*
- *be flexible at each feed, but check that the intake is adequate by measuring the daily weight gain.*

Experience shows that mothers learn this method quickly. Moreover, it has an advantage over other methods since no utensils are required, thus ensuring good hygiene. It is not possible, however, to assess the amount of milk given, especially at the beginning, when it could be too small for the baby's needs. Later, it can be assumed to be adequate as long as the baby is gaining weight (see below). The method has, however, not been assessed systematically and compared to other methods.

Cup-feeding

Cups and other traditional utensils such as the "paladai" in India[53] can be used to feed even very small babies, as long as they swallow the milk.[59,60] For details of cup-feeding techniques, see the WHO breastfeeding counselling course (pp. 340-344).[19]

Mothers can easily learn this technique and feed their babies with adequate amounts of milk. Cup-feeding presents a few advantages over bottle-feeding since it does not interfere with suckling at the breast; a cup is easily cleaned with soap and water, if boiling is not possible, and enables the baby to control his own intake. At first, the mother may prefer to take the baby out of the kangaroo position.

Syringe or dropper-feeding

The technique is similar to that for expressing breast milk in baby's mouth: measure the required amount of breast milk in a cup and pour it directly into the baby's mouth with a regular or special spoon, syringe or dropper. Some more milk is given once the baby has swallowed the given amount. Spoon-feeding takes longer than cup-feeding and spillage can be substantial. Feeding with syringes and droppers is not faster than cup-feeding. Moreover, syringes and droppers are more difficult to clean and more expensive.

Bottle-feeding

This is the least preferred feeding method and is not recommended. It may hinder breathing and oxygenation[61, 62] and it interferes with suckling. Bottles and teats must be sterilized in institutions, and boiled at home.

Tube-feeding

Tube-feeding is used when the baby cannot yet swallow, or coordinate swallowing and breathing, or tires too easily and does not get enough milk. While the health worker inserts the tube and prepares the syringe or dropper, mother can let the baby suck her breast.

The baby can be tube-fed in the kangaroo position.

How to insert a tube

- Take the baby out of the kangaroo position, wrap her in a warm cloth and place her on a warm surface;
- insert the tube through the baby's mouth rather than the nose: small babies breathe through the nose and the tube placed in the nostrils may obstruct breathing;
- use No. 5 to No. 8 French gauge short feeding tubes, depending on the size of the infant;
- measure and mark the distance from the mouth to the ear and to the lower tip of the sternum on the tube with a felt pen;
- pass the tube through the mouth into the stomach until the felt pen mark reaches the lips; baby's breathing should be normal with the tube in place;
- secure the tube to the infant's face with a tape;
- replace the tube every 24-72 hours. Keep it closed or pinched while removing it to avoid dripping fluid into the baby's throat.

How to prepare and use the syringe

- Determine the amount of milk for the feed (Table 3);
- choose the corresponding size syringe;
- remove the piston from the syringe and discard it;
- attach the syringe to the tube;
- pour the required amount of breast milk into the syringe;
- hold the syringe barrel above baby's stomach and let the milk flow by gravity; do not inject the milk;
- observe the baby during feeding for any change in breathing and spilling;
- when feeding is completed close off the tube with a spigot;
- during tube-feeding baby can suck the breast or the mother's finger (Fig.8).

As soon as the baby shows signs of readiness for oral feeding (breastfeeding or cup, spoon, syringe, or dropper-feeding), feed at first once or twice a day, while the baby is still mostly fed through a tube. Gradually reduce tube feeds and remove the tube when the baby takes at least three consecutive feeds of breast milk by cup.

Quantity and frequency

Frequency of feeding will depend on the quantity of milk the baby tolerates per feed and the required daily amount. As a guide, the amount per feed for small newborn preterm babies should be steadily increased as follows:

❖ *up to day 5 slowly increase the total amount and the amount per feed, to help the newborn infant get used to enteral feeding;*
❖ *after day 5 steadily increase the quantity to achieve the amount required for the baby's age as indicated in Tables 2 and 3;*
❖ *by day 14 the baby should take 200ml/kg/day, which is the amount required for steady growth.*

Table 3 shows the approximate amount and number of feeds required as the baby grows older. Avoid overfeeding or feeding too rapidly to lessen the risk of milk aspiration or abdominal distension.

Very small babies should be fed every two hours, larger babies every three hours. If necessary, wake mother and baby during the day and night to ensure regular feeding.

Table 2. Amount of milk (or fluid) needed per day by birth weight and age								
Birth weight	Feed every	Day 1	Day 2	Day 3	Day 4	Day 5	Days 6-13	Day 14
1000-1499g ≥1500 g	2 hours 3 hours	60 ml/kg	80 ml/kg	90 ml/kg	100 ml/kg	110 ml/kg	120-180 ml/kg	180-200 ml/kg

Table 3. Approximate amount of breast milk needed per feed by birth weight and age								
Birth weight	Number of feeds	Day 1	Day 2	Day 3	Day 4	Day 5	Days 6-13	Day 14
1000g	12	5 ml/kg	7 ml/kg	8 ml/kg	9 ml/kg	10 ml/kg	11-16 ml/kg	17 ml/kg
1250g	12	6 ml/kg	8 ml/kg	9 ml/kg	11 ml/kg	12 ml/kg	14-19 ml/kg	21 ml/kg
1500g	8	12 ml/kg	15 ml/kg	17 ml/kg	19 ml/kg	21 ml/kg	23-33 ml/kg	35 ml/kg
1750g	8	14 ml/kg	18 ml/kg	20 ml/kg	22 ml/kg	24 ml/kg	26-42 ml/kg	45 ml/kg
2000g	8	15 ml/kg	20 ml/kg	23 ml/kg	25 ml/kg	28 ml/kg	30-45 ml/kg	50 ml/kg

Transition from an alternative feeding method to exclusive breastfeeding may occur earlier in larger babies and much later in very small babies and may take a week. Encourage mother to start breastfeeding as soon as the baby shows signs of readiness. At the beginning the baby may not suckle long enough but even short sucking stimulates milk production and helps the baby to "practice". Keep reassuring the mother and helping her with breastfeeding the baby. As the baby grows, gradually replace scheduled feeding with feeding on demand.

When the baby moves on to exclusive breastfeeding and measuring the amount of milk intake is not possible, weight gain remains the only way to assess whether feeding is adequate.

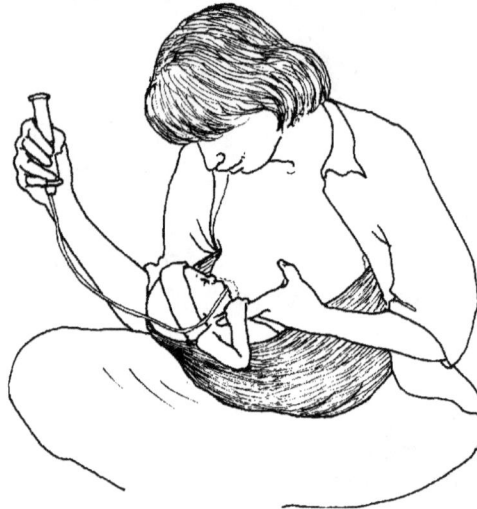

Fig.8   Tube-feeding in KMC

If the mother is HIV-positive and chooses replacement feeding, suggest using cup-feeding. For further information on this issue, please refer to HIV and infant feeding counselling course.[20]

4.8   Monitoring growth

Weight

Weigh small babies daily and check weight gain to assess first the adequacy of fluid intake and then growth. Small babies lose weight at first, immediately after birth: weight loss of up to 10% in the first few days of life has been considered acceptable. After the initial weight loss, newborn babies will slowly regain birth weight, usually between 7 and 14 days after birth. After that babies should be gaining weight, a little at the beginning, more later on. No weight loss is acceptable though after this initial period. Good weight gain is considered a sign of good health, poor weight gain is a serious concern. There is no upper limit for weight gain for breastfed infants, but the lower limit should be no less than 15g/kg/day.

> *Adequate daily weight gain from the second week of life is15g/kg/day. Approximate weight gains for different post-menstrual ages are given below:*
>
> ❖ *20g/day up to 32 weeks of post-menstrual age, corresponding approximately to 150-200g/week;*
> ❖ *25g/day from 33 to 36 weeks of post-menstrual age, corresponding approximately to 200-250g/week;*
> ❖ *30g/day from 37 to 40 weeks of post-menstrual age, corresponding approximately to 250-300g/week.*

There are no universally accepted recommendations regarding frequency of growth monitoring for LBW and preterm infants. There is no universal reference chart for plotting the postnatal weight gain of those babies but intrauterine growth charts by week of gestation, with percentiles or standard deviations, are used instead.

It is not known whether an extrauterine growth similar to the one the preterm infant would have had in utero is an appropriate criterion for monitoring postnatal weight gain. It seems reasonable, however, to aim for a weight of at least 2500g or more by the 40th week of post-menstrual age.

The following recommendations are based on experience

- *Weigh babies once a day; more frequent weighing might upset the baby and be a cause of anxiety and concern for the mother. Once the baby has started gaining weight, weigh every second day for a week and then once weekly until the baby has reached full term (40 weeks or 2500g);*
- *weigh the baby in the same way every time, i.e. naked, with the same calibrated scales (with 10g intervals if possible), placing a clean warm towel on the scales to avoid cooling the infant;*
- *weigh the baby in a warm environment;*
- *if you have a local weight chart showing the expected intrauterine growth, plot the weight on the graph to monitor growth.*

Growth monitoring, especially for daily weight gain, requires accurate and precise scales and a standardized weighing technique. Spring scales are not precise enough for frequent monitoring of weight gain when weight is low, and may lead to wrong decisions. Analogue maternity hospital scales (with 10g intervals) are the best alternative. If such accurate and precise scales are not available, do not weigh KMC infants daily but rely on weekly weighing for growth monitoring. Weight is recorded on a weight chart and weight gain is assessed daily or weekly.

Head circumference

Measure head circumference weekly. Once baby is gaining weight, head circumference will increase by between 0.5 and 1cm per week. For adequacy of head growth refer to national anthropometric standards.

Alternative methods for monitoring growth

Alternative methods, such as measuring baby's length, and chest and arm circumference, are less useful for growth monitoring and are not recommended for the following reasons:
- length is less reliable than weight. It increases more slowly and does not help to make decisions about feeding or illness;
- surrogates, such as chest and arm circumference, have been proposed to assess size at birth and as a tool to evaluate the need for special care.[63, 64] Their effectiveness for growth monitoring in LBW and preterm infants has not yet been assessed.

4.9 Inadequate weight gain

If weight gain is inadequate for several days, first assess the feeding technique, frequency, duration and schedule, and check that night feeds are given. Advise the mother to increase the frequency of feeds or to feed on demand. Encourage her to drink fluids when thirsty.

Then look for other conditions as possible reasons for poor weight gain:

- ❖ *oral thrush (white patches in the mouth) can interfere with feeding. Treat the baby by giving her an oral suspension of nystatin (100,000 IU/ml); use a dropper to apply 1ml in the oral mucosa and paint the mother's nipples after each feed until the lesions heal. Treat for 7 days;*
- ❖ *rhinitis is quite disturbing for the baby because it interferes with feeding. Nasal drops of normal saline solution in each nostril before each feed may help to relieve nasal obstruction;*
- ❖ *urinary tract infection is a possible insidious cause. Investigate if the baby fails to grow without obvious reasons. Treat according to national/local treatment guidelines;*
- ❖ *severe bacterial infection can initially manifest itself with poor weight gain and poor feeding. If a previously healthy baby becomes unwell and stops feeding, consider this as a serious danger sign. Investigate for infection and treat according to national/local treatment guidelines.*

Other causes of failure to gain weight include patent ductus arteriosus and other diseases that may be difficult to diagnose in settings with scarce resources. Refer the baby who fails to gain weight after the exclusion or treatment of the above common causes to a higher level of care, for further investigation and treatment.

If a mother's breast milk supply is reduced and does not satisfy baby's needs, she must increase it. This often happens where there is a breastfeeding difficulty: baby is not suckling well, the mother has been away or sick and stopped feeding her baby (on increasing breast milk and relactation see the WHO breastfeeding counselling course, pp 348-358,[19] and the WHO document *Relactation: A review of experience and recommendations for practice*[65]). This should be the first step before turning to other methods.

Lactogogues

Herbal teas obtained from sesame, fenugreek, fennel, cumin, basil and aniseed have not been proven effective in increasing breast milk production. Beer and other alcoholic drinks used in some cultures to increase lactation should be discouraged since alcohol in breast milk is dangerous for babies.[66, 67] Domperidone can help increase milk supply. It could be used as a supportive procedure and only after all other effective methods for improving milk production have been tried out. Always follow national guidelines.

If despite all these efforts the baby is not gaining weight, consider supplementing breastfeeding with preterm formula, given by cup after each feed. To prepare formula milk follow the instructions on the box.

Do not make important decisions about formula supplementation on the basis of daily weight, since this is subject to large variations. Only weight change over a few days, or weekly weight gain, is a good basis for such decisions.

Discuss with the mother whether this is a feasible, affordable and safe option that will be available for several months. Show her how to prepare it and give it safely. Follow the instructions on the package. Return to exclusive breastfeeding as soon as possible after the infant has gained weight for some time. Monitor more closely the health and growth of small infants fed or supplemented with formula since they are more exposed than breastfed babies to infection and malnutrition. Try, if at all possible, not to discharge a small baby with formula supplements.

Ensure that the facility follows the rules prescribed by the *International Code of Marketing of Breast-milk Substitutes*, issued by WHO.[68]

4.10 Preventive treatment

Small babies are born without sufficient stores of micronutrients. Preterm babies, irrespective of weight, should receive iron and folic acid supplementation from the second month of life until one year of chronological age. The recommended daily dose of iron is 2mg/kg body weight/day.

- Explain to the mother that:
  - iron is essential for baby's health and growth;
  - the baby needs to take iron regularly: at the same time every day, after breastfeeding;
  - baby's stools may become darker, which is normal.
- Explore her concerns.

4.11 Stimulation

All infants need love and care to flourish, but very preterm babies need even more attention to be able to develop normally since they have been deprived of an ideal intrauterine environment for weeks or even months. They are instead exposed to too much light, noise and painful stimuli during their initial care. KMC is an ideal method since the baby is rocked and cuddled, and listens to the mother's voice while she goes about her everyday activities. Fathers too can provide such an environment. Health workers have an important role to play in encouraging mothers and fathers to express their emotions and love to their babies.

However, if the baby has other problems due to preterm birth or its complications, additional treatment may be necessary. Guidance on such treatment can be found in standard textbooks or in the WHO manual *Managing newborn problems. A guide for doctors, nurses and midwives*.[56]

4.12 Discharge

Discharge means letting the mother and baby go home. Their own environment, however, could be very different from the KMC unit at the facility, where they were surrounded by supportive staff. They will continue to need support even though this will not have to be as intensive and frequent. The time of discharge may therefore vary depending on the size of the baby, bed availability, home conditions and accessibility of follow-up care. Usually, a KMC baby can be discharged from the hospital when the following criteria are met:

- ❖ *the baby's general health is good and there is no concurrent disease such as apnoea or infection;*
- ❖ *he is feeding well, and is exclusively or predominantly breastfed;*
- ❖ *he is gaining weight (at least 15g/kg/day for at least three consecutive days);*

❖ his temperature is stable in the KMC position (within the normal range for at least three consecutive days);

❖ the mother is confident in caring for the baby and is able to come regularly for follow-up visits.

These criteria are usually met by the time the baby weighs more than 1500g.

The home environment is also very important for the successful outcome of KMC. The mother should go back to a warm, smoke-free home and should have support for everyday household tasks.

Where there are no follow-up services and the hospital is far away, mother and baby should be discharged later.

Immunize the baby according to national policy and give enough iron/folate tablets to last until the follow-up visit. Fill in the home-based baby's record. Ensure that the mother knows:

❖ how to apply skin-to-skin contact until baby shows signs of discomfort;

❖ how to dress the baby, when he is not in kangaroo position, to keep him warm at home;

❖ how to bath the baby and keep him warm after the bath;

❖ how to respond to baby's needs such as increasing the duration of skin-to-skin contact if he has cold hands and feet or low temperature at night;

❖ how to breastfeed the baby during the day and night according to instructions;

❖ when and where to return for follow-up visits (schedule the first visit and give the mother written/pictorial instructions for the above issues);

❖ how to recognize danger signs;

❖ where to seek care urgently if danger signs appear;

❖ when to wean the baby from KMC.

She should return immediately to hospital, or go to another appropriate provider, if the baby:

   ❖   stops feeding, is not feeding well, or vomits;

   ❖   becomes restless and irritable, lethargic or unconscious;

   ❖   has fever (body temperature above 37.5°C);

   ❖   is cold (hypothermia - body temperature below 36.5°C) despite rewarming;

   ❖   has convulsions;

   ❖   has difficulty breathing;

   ❖   has diarrhoea;

   ❖   shows any other worrying sign.

Tell the mother that it is always better to seek help, if in doubt: when caring for small infants it is better to seek care too often than to disregard important symptoms.

Early discharge becomes a goal for the mother as she gains confidence in her ability to care for her baby. A baby can be discharged earlier if the following criteria are met:

❖ adequate information on home care is given at discharge to mothers and their families, preferably as written and pictorial instructions;

❖ mothers have received instructions on danger signs, and know when and where to seek care.

4.13 KMC at home and routine follow-up

Ensure follow-up for the mother and the baby, either at your facility or with a skilled provider near the baby's home. The smaller the baby is at discharge, the earlier and more frequent follow-up visits he will need. If the baby is discharged in accordance with the above criteria, the following suggestions will be valid in most circumstances:
    – two follow-up visits per week until 37 weeks of post-menstrual age;
    – one follow-up visit per week after 37 weeks.

The content of the visit may vary according to mother's and baby's needs; check the following, however, at each follow-up visit:

KMC

Duration of skin-to-skin contact, position, clothing, body temperature, support for the mother and the baby. Is the baby showing signs of intolerance? Is it time to wean the baby from KMC (usually at around 40 weeks of post-menstrual age, or just before)? If not, encourage the mother and family to continue KMC as much as possible.

Breastfeeding

Is it exclusive? If yes, praise the mother and encourage her to continue. If not, advise her on how to increase breastfeeding and decrease supplements or other fluids. Ask and look for any problem and provide support. If the baby is taking formula supplements or other foods, check their safety and adequacy; make sure that the family has the necessary supply.

Growth

Weigh the baby and check weight gain in the last period. If weight gain is adequate, i.e. at least 15g/kg/day on average, praise the mother. If it is inadequate, ask and look for possible problems, causes and solutions; these are generally related to feeding or illness. To check adequate daily weight gain please refer to box on page 37.

Illness

Ask and look for any signs of illness, reported by the mother or not. Manage any illness according to your local protocols and guidelines. In case of non-exclusive breastfeeding, ask and look particularly for signs of nutritional or digestive problems.

Drugs

Give a sufficient supply of drugs, if needed, to last until the next follow-up visit.

Immunization

Check that the local immunization schedule is being followed.

Mother's concerns

Ask the mother about any other problem, including personal, household, and social problems. Try to help her find the best solution for all of them.

Next follow-up visit

Always schedule or confirm the next visit. Do not miss the opportunity, if time allows, to check and advise on hygiene, and to reinforce the mother's awareness of danger signs that need prompt care.

Special follow-up visits

If these are required for other medical or somatic problems, encourage the mother to attend them and help her if needed.

Routine child care

Encourage the mother to attend routine child care once the baby reaches 2500g or 40 weeks of post-menstrual age.

References

1   *Low birth weight. A tabulation of available information.* Geneva, World Health Organization, 1992 (WHO/MCH/92.2).

2   de Onis M, Blossner M, Villar J. Levels and patterns of intrauterine growth retardation in developing countries. *European Journal of Clinical Nutrition*, 1998, 52(Suppl.1):S5-S15.

3   *Essential newborn care. Report of a Technical Working Group (Trieste 25-29 April 1994).* Geneva, World Health Organization, 1996 (WHO/FRH/MSM/96.13).

4   Ashworth A. Effects of intrauterine growth retardation on mortality and morbidity in infants and young children. *European Journal of Clinical Nutrition*, 1998, 52(Suppl.1):S34-S41; discussion: S41-42.

5   Murray CJL, Lopez AD, eds. *Global burden of disease: a comprehensive assessment of mortality and disability from diseases, injuries and risk factors in 1990 and projected to 2020.* Boston, Harvard School of Public Health, 1996 (Global burden of disease and injuries series, vol. 1).

6   Gulmezoglu M, de Onis M, Villar J. Effectiveness of interventions to prevent or treat impaired fetal growth. *Obstetrical & Gynecological Survey*, 1997, 52:139-149.

7   Kramer MS. Socioeconomic determinants of intrauterine growth retardation. *European Journal of Clinical Nutrition*, 1998, 52(Suppl.1):S29-S32; discussion: S32-33.

8   McCormick MC. The contribution of low birth weight to infant mortality and childhood morbidity. *The New England Journal of Medicine*, 1985, 312:82-90.

9   Rey ES, Martinez HG. Manejo racional del niño prematuro. In: Universidad Nacional, *Curso de Medicina Fetal*, Bogotá, Universidad Nacional, 1983.

10 *Thermal control of the newborn: A practical guide.* Maternal Health and Safe Motherhood Programme. Geneva, World Health Organization, 1993 (WHO/FHE/MSM/93.2).

11 Shiau SH, Anderson GC. Randomized controlled trial of kangaroo care with fullterm infants: effects on maternal anxiety, breastmilk maturation, breast engorgement, and breast-feeding status. Paper presented at the International Breastfeeding Conference, Australia's Breastfeeding Association, Sydney, October 23-25, 1997.

12 Cattaneo A, *et al.* Recommendations for the implementation of kangaroo mother care for low birthweight infants. *Acta Paediatrica*, 1998, 87:440-445.

13 Cattaneo A, *et al.* Kangaroo mother care in low-income countries. *Journal of Tropical Pediatrics*, 1998, 44:279-282.

14 Bergman NJ, Jürisoo LA. The "kangaroo-method" for treating low birth weight babies in a developing country. *Tropical Doctor*, 1994, 24:57-60.

15 Lincetto O, Nazir AI, Cattaneo A. Kangaroo Mother Care with limited resources. *Journal of Tropical Pediatrics*, 2000, 46:293-295.

16 Anderson GC. Current knowledge about skin-to-skin (kangaroo) care for preterm infants. *Journal of Perinatology*, 1991, 11:216-226.

17 Christensson K, *et al.* Randomised study of skin-to-skin versus incubator care for rewarming low-risk hypothermic neonates. *The Lancet*, 1998, 352:1115.

18 Shekelle PG. Clinical guidelines: Developing guidelines. *British Medical Journal*, 1999, 318:593-596.

19 *Breastfeeding counselling: A training course - Trainer's guide.* Geneva, World Health Organization, 1993 (WHO/CDR/93.4). Also available from UNICEF (UNICEF/NUT/93.2).

20 *HIV and infant feeding counselling: A training course - Trainer's guide.* Geneva, World Health Organization, 2000 (WHO/FCH/CAH/00.3). Also available from UNICEF (UNICEF/PD/NUT/00-4) or UNAIDS (UNAIDS/99.58).

21 Charpak N, Ruiz-Pelaez JG, Figueroa de Calume Z. Current knowledge of kangaroo mother intervention. *Current Opinion in Pediatrics*, 1996, 8:108-112.

22 Ludington-Hoe SM, Swinth JY. Developmental aspects of kangaroo care. *Journal of Obstetric, Gynecologic, and Neonatal Nursing*, 1996, 25:691-703.

23 Conde-Agudelo A, Diaz-Rosello JL, Belizan JM. Kangaroo mother care to reduce morbidity and mortality in low birth weight infants. *Cochrane Library*, Issue 2, 2002.

24 Sloan NL, *et al*. Kangaroo mother method: randomised controlled trial of an alternative method of care for stabilised low-birthweight infants. *The Lancet*, 1994, 344:782-785.

25 Charpak N, *et al*. Kangaroo mother versus traditional care for newborn infants ≤ 2000 grams: a randomized controlled trial. *Pediatrics*, 1997, 100:682-688.

26 Cattaneo A, *et al*. Kangaroo mother care for low birthweight infants: a randomised controlled trial in different settings. *Acta Paediatrica*, 1998, 87:976-985.

27 Kambarami RA, Chidede O, Kowo DT. Kangaroo care versus incubator care in the management of well preterm infants: a pilot study. *Annals of Tropical Paediatrics*, 1998, 18:81-86.

28 Whitelaw A, Sleath K. Myth of marsupial mother: home care of very low birth weight infants in Bogotá, Colombia. *The Lancet*, 1985, 1:1206-1208.

29 Charpak N, *et al*. Kangaroo-mother programme: an alternative way of caring for low birth weight infants? One year mortality in a two-cohort study. *Pediatrics*, 1994, 94:804-810.

30 Anderson GC, *et al*. Birth-associated fatigue in 34-36 week premature infants: rapid recovery with very early skin-to-skin (kangaroo) care. *Journal of Obstetric, Gynecologic, and Neonatal Nursing*, 1999, 28:94-103.

31 Lincetto O, *et al*. Impact of season and discharge weight on complications and growth of kangaroo mother care treated low birthweight infants in Mozambique. *Acta Paediatrica*, 1998, 87:433-439.

32 Schmidt E, Wittreich G. Care of the abnormal newborn: a random controlled trial study of the "kangaroo method" of care of low birth weight newborns. In: *Consensus Conference on Appropriate Technology Following Birth, Trieste, 7-11 October 1986*. WHO Regional Office for Europe.

33 Whitelaw A, *et al*. Skin-to-skin contact for very low birth weight infants and their mothers. *Archives of Disease in Childhood*, 1988, 63:1377-1381.

34 Wahlberg V, Affonso D, Persson B. A retrospective, comparative study using the kangaroo method as a complement to the standard incubator care. *European Journal of Public Health*, 1992, 2:34-37.

35 Syfrett EB, *et al*. Early and virtually continuous kangaroo care for lower-risk preterm infants: effect on temperature, breast-feeding, supplementation and weight. In: *Proceedings of the Biennial Conference of the Council of Nurse Researchers*. Washington, DC, American Nurses Association, 1993.

36 Blaymore-Bier JA, *et al*. Comparison of skin-to-skin contact with standard contact in low birth weight infants who are breastfed. *Archives of Pediatrics & Adolescent Medicine*, 1996, 150:1265-1269.

37 Hurst NM, *et al*. Skin-to-skin holding in the neonatal intensive care unit influences maternal milk volume. *Journal of Perinatology*, 1997, 17:213-217.

38 Christensson K. Fathers can effectively achieve heat conservation in healthy newborn infants. *Acta Paediatrica*, 1996, 85:1354-1360.

39 Ludington-Hoe SM, *et al*. Selected physiologic measures and behavior during paternal skin contact with Colombian preterm infants. *Journal of Developmental Physiology*, 1992, 18:223-232.

40 Acolet D, Sleath K, Whitelaw A. Oxygenation, heart rate and temperature in very low birth weight infants during skin-to-skin contact with their mothers. *Acta Paediatrica Scandinavica*, 1989, 78: 189-193.

41 de Leeuw R, *et al*. Physiologic effects of kangaroo care in very small preterm infants. *Biology of the Neonate*, 1991, 59:149-155.

42 Fischer C, *et al*. Cardiorespiratory stability of premature boys and girls during kangaroo care. *Early Human Development*, 1998, 52:145-153.

43 Anderson GC, Wood CE, Chang HP. Self-regulatory mothering vs. nursery routine care postbirth: effect on salivary cortisol and interactions with gender, feeding, and smoking. *Infant Behavior and Development*, 1998, 21:264.

44 Christensson K, *et al*. Temperature, metabolic adaptation and crying in healthy full-term newborns cared for skin-to-skin or in a cot. *Acta Paediatrica*, 1992, 81:488-493.

45 Christensson K, *et al*. Separation distress call in the human infant in the absence of maternal body contact. *Acta Paediatrica*, 1995, 84:468-473.

46 Affonso D, Wahlberg V, Persson B. Exploration of mother's reactions to the kangaroo method of prematurity care. *Neonatal Network*, 1989, 7:43-51.

47 Affonso D, *et al.* Reconciliation and healing for mothers through skin-to-skin contact provided in an American tertiary level intensive care nursery. *Neonatal Network*, 1993,12:25-32.

48 Legault M, Goulet C. Comparison of kangaroo and traditional methods of removing preterm infants from incubators. *Journal of Obstetric, Gynecologic, and Neonatal Nursing*, 1995, 24:501-506.

49 Bell EH, Geyer J, Jones L. A structured intervention improves breast-feeding success for ill or preterm infants. *American Journal of Maternal and Child Nursing*, 1995, 20:309-314.

50 Tessier R, *et al.* Kangaroo mother care and the bonding hypothesis. *Pediatrics*, 1998, 102:390-391.

51 Hylander MA, Strobino DM, Dhanireddy R. Human milk feedings and infection among very low birth weight infants. *Pediatrics*, 1998, 102:E38.

52 Schanler RJ, Shulman RJ, Lau C. Feeding strategies for premature infants: beneficial outcomes of feeding fortified human milk versus preterm formula. *Pediatrics*, 1999, 103:1150-1157.

53 Malhotra N, *et al.* A controlled trial of alternative methods of oral feeding in neonates. *Early Human Development*, 1999, 54:29-38.

54 Sontheimer D, *et al.* Pitfalls in respiratory monitoring of premature infants during kangaroo care. *Archives of Disease in Childhood*, 1995, 72:F115-117.

55 Lubchenco LO, *et al.* Intrauterine growth as estimated from live born birth weight data at 24 to 42 weeks of gestation. *Pediatrics*, 1963, 32:793-800.

56 *Managing newborn problems. A guide for doctors, nurses and midwives.* Geneva, World Health Organization (in press).

57 Jenni OG, *et al.* Effect of nursing in the head elevated tilt position (15 degrees) on the incidence of bradycardic and hypoxemic episodes in preterm infants. *Pediatrics*, 1997, 100:622-625.

58 Ludington-Hoe SM, Hadeed AJ, Anderson GC. Physiologic responses to skin-to-skin contact in hospitalized premature infants. *Journal of Perinatology*, 1991, 11:19-24.

59 Gupta A, Khanna K, Chattree S. Cup feeding: an alternative to bottle feeding in a neonatal intensive care unit. *Journal of Tropical Pediatrics*, 1999, 45:108-110.

60 Lang S, Lawrence CJ, Orme RL. Cup feeding: an alternative method of infant feeding. *Archives of Disease in Childhood*, 1994, 71:365-369.

61 Bier JB, *et al.* Breast-feeding of very low birth weight infants. *Journal of Pediatrics*, 1993, 123:773-778.

62 Poets CF, Langner MU, Bohnhorst B. Effects of bottle feeding and two different methods of gavage feeding on oxygenation and breathing patterns in preterm infants. *Acta Paediatrica*, 1997, 86:419-423.

63 *Birth weight surrogates: The relationship between birth weight, arm and chest circumference.* Geneva, World Health Organization, 1987.

64 Diamond JD, *et al.* The relationship between birth weight and arm and chest circumference in Egypt. *Journal of Tropical Pediatrics*, 1991, 37:323-6.

65 *Relactation: A review of experience and recommendations for practice.* Geneva, World Health Organization, 1998 (WHO/CHS/CAH/98.14).

66 Mennella JA, Gerrish CJ. Effects of exposure to alcohol in mother's milk on infant sleep. *Pediatrics*, 1998, 101:E2.

67 Rosti L, *et al.* Toxic effects of a herbal tea mixture in two newborns. *Acta Paediatrica*, 1994, 83:683.

68 *International code of marketing of breast-milk substitutes.* Geneva, World Health Organization, 1981 (HA34/1981/REC/1, Annex 3).

Annexes

I Records and indicators

Clinical records for hospital and follow-up care of small babies vary from place to place and according to the level of care offered to LBW and preterm infants. Essential information on KMC, when this is part of the care programme, must also be recorded. The following additional information should be recorded daily:

- ❖ For the baby hospital record:
  - when KMC began (date, weight and age);
  - condition of the baby;
  - details on duration and frequency of skin-to-skin contact;
  - whether the mother is hospitalized or is coming from home;
  - predominant feeding method;
  - observations about lactation and feeding;
  - daily weight gain;
  - episodes of illness, other conditions or complications;
  - the drugs baby is receiving;
  - details on discharge: condition of the baby, maternal readiness, conditions at home that make discharge possible; date, age, weight and post-menstrual age at discharge; feeding method and instructions for follow-up (where, when and how frequently).

Mother should be given a discharge letter summarizing the course of hospitalization and instructions for home care, medication and follow-up. It is also necessary to record whether the baby was transferred to another institution or died.

- ❖ The follow-up record should contain, besides the usual data on the baby, the following information:
  - when the baby was first seen (date, age, weight and post-menstrual age);
  - feeding method;
  - daily duration of skin-to-skin contact;
  - any concerns mother may have;
  - whether baby has to be or has been readmitted to hospital;
  - when mother stopped skin-to-skin contact (date, age of the baby, weight, post-menstrual age, reasons for stopping and feeding method at weaning);
  - other important remarks.

If the follow-up care is provided at the facility where the baby was hospitalized, the hospital record and the follow-up record should be a single document. If this cannot be done, the two records must be linked by an identification number. The records can obviously be used to develop an electronic database. The follow-up record presented in this annex is derived from those used by KMC programmes in some countries.

An example of how information on KMC can be added to the follow-up record:

Date of visit	.. /.. /....	.. /.. /....	.. /.. /....	.. /.. /....	.. /.. /....	.. /.. /....	.. /.. /....	.. /.. /....
Age								
Weight weight gain								
Feeding method								
Average daily duration of skin-to-skin contact								
Complaints								
Readmission to hospital								
Weaned Date Age (in days) Post-menstrual age Weight	Reasons for weaning and other comments							

These data will provide basic information for daily baby care and process and outcome indicators for programme monitoring.

❖ When KMC forms part of a care programme for small babies it is important to know the following:

- the number of small babies (<2000g and/or <34 weeks) treated and the proportion receiving KMC;
- mean age at start of KMC (stratified by weight and gestational age at birth, and weight and post-menstrual age when starting);
- type of KMC (predominant or partial);
- mean duration of KMC (in days);
- mean weight gain during KMC in institution and at home;
- mean age of weaning from KMC (stratified by weight and gestational age at birth, and weight and post-menstrual age when starting);
- feeding method for babies at weaning from KMC (exclusively/partly breastfed, or not breastfed);
- proportion of babies needing hospitalization during home KMC;
- death rate during KMC, at institution and at home.

II Birth weight and gestational age

At different gestational ages birth weight can vary by about one kilogram; at a given weight babies can be of different gestational ages.

Table 4. Mean birth weights (g) with 10th and 90th percentiles by gestational age			
Gestational age	Mean birth weight	10th percentile	90th percentile
28	1200	900	1500
29	1350	1000	1650
30	1500	1100	1750
31	1650	1200	2000
32	1800	1300	2350
33	2000	1500	2500
34	2250	1750	2750
35	2500	2000	3000
36	2750	2250	3250
37	3000	2450	3500
38	3200	2650	3700
39	3350	2800	3900
40	3500	3000	4100

III Constraints

KMC has been included in national guidelines for the care of LBW and preterm infants, and successfully implemented in many countries. Experience shows that the main problems, obstacles and constraints fall under four categories: policy, implementation, communication and feeding. Some possible solutions are suggested in Table 5.

Table 5. Implementing KMC	
Problems, obstacles and constraints	*Possible solutions*
Policy	
• Lack of plans, policies, guidelines, protocols, manuals • Lack of institutional, academic and professional support • Lack of adequate training and continuous education • Risk of an isolated and vertical programme • Poor access to evidence, literature and documentation • Legal problems (e.g. KMC not included in the interventions financed by the health care system)	• Development of plans, policies, guidelines, protocols, manuals • Establishing links with ministries, medical schools, agencies and organizations; advocacy work • Establishing basic, post-graduate and in-service courses • Integration with existing programmes • Creation of local and regional libraries; links with main documentation centres • Proposing changes to existing laws, rules and regulations; involving mothers and families
Implementation	
• Resistance of managers, administrators and health workers • Poor facilities, equipment, supplies, organization, lack of time • Cultural problems: misguided beliefs, attitudes, practices • Apparent initial increase of workload • Redistribution of tasks, multidisciplinary approach • Resistance of mothers and families • Lack of monitoring and evaluation	• Adequate information on effectiveness, safety, feasibility and cost • Improving structure and organization, procurement of basic equipment; ensuring supplies • Appropriate training and information strategies, community participation • Introducing changes step-by-step • Writing new job descriptions, encouraging team work and frequent joint review of problems • Hospital and community support groups • Gathering, analysing and discussing standard data
Communication	
• Mothers and families unaware of KMC • Poor communication and support in hospital and during follow-up • Inadequate community and family support • Hostility of politicians and other health professionals	• Adequate information in the antenatal period and at the referral facility • Improving communication and support skills of health workers • Community meetings, mass media, hot lines • Articles, newsletters, interest groups, testimonies
Feeding	
• Low rate of exclusive breastfeeding after long separation of infants from mothers • Difficult growth monitoring, lack of adequate standards • Inadequate growth despite good implementation of breastfeeding guidelines • High prevalence of HIV-positive mothers	• Reducing separation as much as possible; implementation of feeding guidelines • Accurate scales, appropriate growth charts, clear instructions • Good skills for assessing breastfeeding and alternative feeding methods • Voluntary counselling and testing of parents; infant feeding counselling, appropriate replacement feeding for preterm infants; safe alternatives to breast milk; pasteurisers